医疗器械注册共性问题
百 问 百 答 2

（中英文版）

国家药品监督管理局医疗器械技术审评中心
组织编写

中国健康传媒集团
中国医药科技出版社

图书在版编目（CIP）数据

医疗器械注册共性问题百问百答 . 2：汉英对照 / 国家药品监督管理局医疗器械技术审评中心组织编写 . — 北京：中国医药科技出版社，2023.7

ISBN 978-7-5214-3961-8

Ⅰ.①医… Ⅱ.①国… Ⅲ.①医疗器械—注册—中国—问题解答—汉、英 Ⅳ.① R197.39-44

中国国家版本馆 CIP 数据核字（2023）第 102312 号

责任编辑 吴思思 张 睿
美术编辑 陈君杞
版式设计 也 在

出版	**中国健康传媒集团** | 中国医药科技出版社
地址	北京市海淀区文慧园北路甲 22 号
邮编	100082
电话	发行：010-62227427　邮购：010-62236938
网址	www.cmstp.com
规格	880×1230mm $\frac{1}{32}$
印张	7
字数	152 千字
版次	2023 年 7 月第 1 版
印次	2023 年 7 月第 1 次印刷
印刷	三河市万龙印装有限公司
经销	全国各地新华书店
书号	ISBN 978-7-5214-3961-8
定价	**40.00 元**

获取新书信息、投稿、为图书纠错，请扫码联系我们。

内容提要

本书由国家药品监督管理局医疗器械技术审评中心组织编写,是一线审评人员实践经验与专家学者的专业化理论知识的有机结合,全面梳理出咨询频率高、咨询次数多、存在问题广的 161 个医疗器械行业审评中的问题,涵盖有源医疗器械、无源医疗器械、体外诊断试剂产品及其他共性问题等四个方面,对审评注册中的技术问题、法规理解等内容,逐一解答,并采用中英文对照方式进行展示。本书适合各级监管部门、审评机构以及从事医疗器械注册申报的行政相对人参考使用。

编委会

前　言

健康是人类最关切的议题、是人类最永恒的追求、是人类最宝贵的财富。医疗器械的安全性和有效性与公众健康和生命安全息息相关。随着新版《医疗器械监督管理条例》的颁布与实施，我国医疗器械法规体系日益完善，先进的监管理念和方法与医疗器械产业相结合，不断促进医疗器械行业的发展。

为响应国家深化简政放权、放管结合、优化服务改革，国家药品监督管理局医疗器械技术审评中心（以下简称"器审中心"）不断完善对外沟通交流渠道，提高行政相对人服务质量。针对咨询频率较高的审评热点问题，器审中心结合我国医疗器械规章制度要求形成共性问题解答，并通过网站、微信公众号等媒介对外发布。第一版《医疗器械注册共性问题百问百答》自2020年出版以来，深受医疗器械注册从业者的广泛好评。在此基础上，器审中心继续组织编写《医疗器械注册共性问题百问百答2》一书。本书梳理近年来出现频率高、咨询次数多、存在问题广的医疗器械行业共性问题，并采用中英文对照方式进行展示，是总结上一版书籍编撰经验的基础上形成的，是一线审评人员实践经验与专家学者的专业化理论知识的有机结合，将对全面提高行业人员能力和素质起到进一步的促进作用。

全书共分四章，第一章至第三章分别为有源医疗器械、无源医疗器械、体外诊断试剂产品技术共性问题，涵盖人工智能医疗器械、动物源性医疗器械、增材制造医疗器械、临床检验仪器等行业关注热点问题和体外诊断试剂产品审评要求和临床试验等相关问题的中英文双解答；第四章为其他技术共性问题，涵盖医疗器械临床评价问题、创新医疗器械审查、技术审评流程，以及其他注册申报资料的相关问题及解答。各章内容均按照不同分类进行排序，涉及相应问题与解答 161 个，适合各级监管部门、审评机构以及从事医疗器械注册申报的行政相对人阅读使用。

由于医疗器械行业涉及学科多、概念广、理论新、技术含量高，本书还需在实践中得到检验，欢迎广大读者提出宝贵的意见和建议。

编　者

2023 年 6 月

目　录

第一章

有源医疗器械产品技术共性问题

1. 问：术中脑电/肌电/诱发电位测量系统等设备的电刺激器和针电极是否可以单独注册？

答：术中脑电/肌电/诱发电位测量系统等设备在使用时通常需要电刺激器、针电极等附件。通常电刺激器和连接使用的设备是一体的，可以和设备一起注册。针电极通常为独立的无菌包装，一次性使用，在医疗器械分类目录中单独作为医疗器械管理，建议单独注册。

2. 问：与放疗系统配合使用的 X 射线图像引导系统，在进行检测时是否需配合放疗系统检测？

答：对于通用型 X 射线图像引导系统，选择有代表性的放疗系统进行兼容性验证，提供验证测试资料，并说明选择测试的放疗系统具有代表性的理由；综述资料中应明确可配合使用的放疗系统的总体要求、接口的类型等信息。

对于专用型 X 射线图像引导系统，需和配合使用的放疗系统应进行验证测试，并提供验证测试资料；综述资料中应明确配合使用的放疗系统的制造商、型号、注册证号（提供注册证复印件）等信息。

3. 问：医用 X 射线诊断设备如适用于儿科人群，针对该特定人群应提交哪些研究资料？

答：由于儿童或新生儿对 X 射线非常敏感，如果行政相对人声称设备适用于儿科人群，应提供降低儿童或新生儿辐射剂量所需采取的措施。如为儿科患者设计自动曝光控制并校准；具有适合婴幼儿的低辐射剂量协议；特殊的滤过系统；低于成年人的辐射入射剂量，曝光限值提示；显示和记录患者剂量信息或剂量指数以及患者其他信息，如年龄、身高和体重（手动输入或自动计算）；具有不用工具即可拆除的滤线栅等。

4. 问：部分有源医疗器械申报时，注册单元内包含可重复使用的附件，这些附件的消毒灭菌资料应关注哪些问题？

答： 对于可重复使用的附件，使用前应保证已消毒或灭菌。说明书中应明确具体的消毒 / 灭菌方法（如使用的消毒剂、消毒或灭菌设备），消毒 / 灭菌周期的重要参数（如时间、温度和压力等）。研究资料中应提供消毒 / 灭菌方法确定的依据、消毒 / 灭菌效果确认资料及推荐的消毒 / 灭菌方法耐受性的研究资料。

如有源医疗器械附件较多，可在消毒灭菌资料中列表说明附件的名称、型号、使用方法、接触人体部位、消毒 / 灭菌方法、验证资料编号等关键信息，提高资料的可读性。

5. 问：牙科光固化机类产品通常含导光元件，导光元件在进行检测时应关注哪些问题？

答： 如果光固化机在临床使用过程中必须配有导光元件，则检测时，光固化机应配合导光元件进行测试，来评估是否符合 YY 0055.1《牙科光固化机第 1 部分：石英钨卤素灯》或 YY 0055.2《牙科光固化机第 2 部分：发光二极管（LED）灯》

中辐射条款 7.2 的要求。检测时选择的导光元件类型或型号应能涵盖申报产品组成中所有的导光元件，或随机文件中明确的可配合使用的所有导光元件。检测报告中应体现导光元件类型或型号。预期使用过程中不需导光元件的光固化机应在正常使用条件下进行测试。

6. 问：有源设备变更注册时，仅功率［包括输入功率和（或）输出功率］发生变化，检测时是否需要做全性能检测？

答： 无需进行全性能检测。行政相对人应分析申报产品具体哪些部件发生变化，在综述资料中对变化情况进行详细描述，研究资料中提供对变化的验证资料。分析变化对产品技术要求中性能指标、电气安全和电磁兼容的影响，对有影响的部分进行检测。

7. 问：X 射线类放射诊断设备用辐射防护附件，是否可以和放射诊断设备一起申报？

答： X 射线类放射诊断设备使用时进行辐射防护的附件，如防辐射衣、防辐射帽、防辐射裙、防辐射围领、医用射线防护眼镜等，用于进行放射诊断时对人体的防护。该类防护附件通常和放射诊断设备无电气连接和物理连接，《医疗器械分类目录》中单独作为医疗器械管理，建议单独申报。不可拆卸的附件除外。

8. 问：软件产品（包括独立软件和软件组件），在确定使用期限时应关注哪些问题？

答： 独立软件的使用期限即软件生存周期时限，通过商业因素予以确定，无需提供验证资料。

软件组件的使用期限与所属医疗器械相同，无需单独体现。专用型独立软件视为软件组件，使用期限要求与独立软件相同，应在所属医疗器械使用期限研究资料中体现。

9. 问：如果申报产品与配合用产品（配合用产品不在注册申报单元内），通过非网线方式（如蓝牙、视频线、存储媒介等）交换数据，是否需要考虑网络安全？

答： 参照《医疗器械网络安全注册审查指导原则》要求，电子数据交换方式包括无线、有线网络，单向、双向数据传输，实时、非实时远程控制控制、存储媒介。

通过非网线方式交换视频数据，属于电子数据交换，应考虑网络安全相应要求。

10. 问：植入式心脏除颤器及同类产品是否需要引用 GB 16174.2《手术植入物有源植入式医疗器械 第 2 部分：心脏起搏器》？

答： 植入式心脏除颤器及同类产品在产品技术要求已引用 GB 16174.1 和 YY 0989.6 的情况下，尽管植入式心脏除颤器具有起搏功能，但因 YY 0989.6 中已充分考虑到了植入式心脏除颤器所具有的起搏功能并作出了相应规定，所以无须引用 GB 16174.2 标准。

11. 问：病人监护仪等含有较多附件的有源医疗器械，提交消毒灭菌资料时应注意哪些问题？

答： 对于含有较多附件的有源医疗器械，因附件较多造成申报资料较多，为便于资料审查，建议提交消毒灭菌资料时，按照申请表结构组成顺序列表说明附件的名称、消毒/灭菌方法、一次性使用/可重复使用、生产企业灭菌/终端用户灭菌等信息。

生产企业灭菌应明确灭菌工艺（方法和参数）和无菌保证水平（SAL），并提供灭菌确认报告。终端用户灭菌应当明确推荐的灭菌工艺（方法和参数）及所推荐的灭菌方法确定的依据；对可耐受两次或多次灭菌的产品，应当提供产品相关推荐的灭菌方法耐受性的研究资料。

如灭菌使用的方法容易出现残留，应当明确残留物信息及采取的处理方法，并提供研究资料。终端用户消毒应当明确推荐的消毒工艺（方法和参数）以及所推荐消毒方法确定的依据。

12. 问：已注册有源产品，结构组成中的充电器输出电流发生变化，标签也相应变化，这种变化是否需要申请变更注册？

答： 应分析变化是否涉及产品技术要求及其他注册证载明

事项内容变化。如涉及，应申请变更注册。如不涉及，应按照企业质量管理体系要求做好相关工作，无需申请变更注册。

13. 问：病人监护仪等含有较多和人体接触附件的有源医疗器械，针对附件进行生物相容性评价时应关注哪些问题？

答： 对于含有较多预期作用于人体的附件（包括直接接触和间接接触）的有源医疗器械，因附件较多造成申报资料较多，为便于资料审查，建议针对附件生物学评价情况分为以下三类：

（1）豁免生物相容性评价的，建议参照《医疗器械生物学评价和审查指南》出具没有发生"四、医疗器械生物安全性重新评价"项下"（一）在下列情况下，制造者应当考虑进行生物安全性重新评价"规定情况的说明性文件。

（2）进行生物相容性评价的，建议参照 GB/T 16886.1《医疗器械生物学评价第 1 部分：风险管理过程中的评价与试验》中系统方法框图所示的风险管理过程中生物学评价程序，对附件进行选择和评价。

（3）进行生物相容性试验的，建议按照 GB/T 16886.1《医疗器械生物学评价第 1 部分：风险管理过程中的评价与试验》附录 A，识别风险评定完整数据组需要补充的数据或试验。

14. 问：病人监护仪等含有较多和人体接触附件的有源医疗器械，准备生物相容性评价资料时应关注哪些问题？

答： 通常病人监护仪的心电、体温、血氧、无创血压、有创血压、呼吸、脑电、麻醉等功能模块均含有若干个和人体接触的附件，申报附件数量较多造成申报资料较多，为便于资料的审查，建议参照如下要求准备生物相容性评价资料：

（1）参照申请表结构组成顺序，按功能模块分类，列表说明和人体接触附件的名称、接触的部位、接触时间、接触性质、生物学评价方式（豁免、评价、试验）和对应的评价资料名称、编号。

（2）进行生物学试验的还应说明生物学测试项目、测试依据、测试结果、测试报告编号等内容。

（3）选取有代表性附件进行测试的，应说明典型型号选取的理由。

15. 问：申报产品所含的脚踏开关通过蓝牙与其他组成部分连接并实现遥控功能，是否需要考虑网络安全？

答：蓝牙遥控功能属于电子数据交换，应考虑网络安全相关风险，参照《医疗器械网络安全注册技术审查指导原则》要求提交相应资料。

16. 问：牙科手机申报注册时是否需要引用 GB 9706.1 和 YY 9706.102 标准？

答：考虑牙科手机和接头的照明供电方式，分为带照明装置式、导光式、无照明式三种方式。带照明装置的结构中含照明光源；导光式结构中不含照明光源，仅含有导光纤维束；无照明式结构既不含照明光源，又不带导光装置。带照明装置的应引用 GB 9706.1 和 YY 9706.102 标准，导光式和无照明式无需引用 GB 9706.1 和 YY 9706.102 标准。

17. 问：已注册 CT 设备的高压发生器增加型号，是否可作为同一注册单元申报？

答： 如果高压发生器增加型号，整机性能实质等同，原则上可作为同一注册单元。例如口腔锥形束 CT 设备的 X 射线组合式机头增加型号的情形，可参照执行。

18. 问：内窥镜手术系统申报注册时，产品结构及组成通常包括哪些部分？

答： 内窥镜手术系统通常也被称为"手术机器人"，在申报注册时产品结构及组成通常包括医生控制台、患者手术平台和影像处理平台，并与三维腹腔内窥镜和手术器械等配合使用。通常与系统不存在物理连接或者电气连接的部件或附件不与该系统一同申报注册，与系统存在物理连接或者电气连接的专用部件或者附件可以与系统一同申报注册也可单独申报注册。对于在临床中共同使用，并且与系统连接的通用设备，例如内窥镜冷光源、高频手术设备等，通常不与该系统作为同一个注册单元申报。

19. 问：通过戊二醛浸泡进行消毒、灭菌的医疗器械，如何评价其残留毒性？

答： 关于戊二醛残留的限值和残留的测试目前没有公认的标准和方法。根据 GB/T 16886.1《医疗器械生物学评价 第 1 部分：风险管理过程中的评价与试验》的规定，总体生物学评价应考虑预期的添加剂、工艺污染物和残留物，如果开展生物学试验的医疗器械样品已按照行政相对人规定的方法进行了戊二醛消毒、灭菌，且试验结果符合生物相容性要求，则认为其残留毒性是可接受的。

除戊二醛外，其他采用化学消毒灭菌剂（例如过氧乙酸、邻苯二甲醛等）进行处理的医疗器械可采用同样的方式来进行残留毒性的评价。

20. 问：有源医疗器械产品组成中通常包含台车，电磁兼容检测时是否需要检测台车？

答： 电磁兼容测试布置中分为落地式设备和台式设备，两者试验布置要求不同，试验结果可能存在差异性。因此，实际使用中如果需要台车，电磁兼容检测应包含台车，按照落地式设备进行检测；如果不需要台车，电磁兼容应按照台式设备进行检测。如果实际使用中二者兼有（即台车为可选配件），则电磁兼容测试中应同时按照落地式设备和台式设备两种试验布置进行检测。

21. 问：一次性使用电子内窥镜、三维内窥镜、胶囊式内窥镜，是否属于《免于临床评价医疗器械目录》的产品？还有哪些内窥镜产品不属于《免于临床评价医疗器械目录》的范围？

答:《免于临床评价医疗器械目录》中所述各内窥镜仅限于常规设计的产品，包括传统的光学内窥镜、纤维内窥镜和电子内窥镜。上述产品均为一体式可重复使用设计，预期与冷光源、摄像装置 / 图像处理器配合使用。

一次性使用的电子内窥镜（包括整体为一次性使用的内窥镜、仅插入部为一次性使用的组合式内窥镜）、三维内窥镜和胶囊式内窥镜，均不属于《免于临床评价医疗器械目录》的产品。此外，内置光源的内窥镜也不属于《免于临床评价医疗器械目录》的范围。

22. 问：产品的行业标准中规定，设备应在交流电压为 220V±22V 范围内正常工作，但申报产品的标称工作电压为 100~240V，与行业标准要求有冲突，应以哪个电压进行测试？

答：首先明确，上述产品的行业标准相关条款考虑因素的出发点，是为了保证产品在中国使用时可能出现电压波动的情况下，仍可正常工作。其次，产品标称的电压范围只是表明可以支持的额定电压，和前面所述的并不是同一层面的问题，两者不存在矛盾。因此，对于问题中所述情况，应按照产品实际设计情况申报注册，产品技术要求中标称电压范围应以实际设计参数 100~240V 为准，进行电气安全和电磁兼容检验时也应按照标称电源参数 100~240V 进行检验；而在对产品的行业标准中此条款进行检验时，按照 220V ± 22V 的电压范围进行检验。

23. 问：医疗器械软件新增临床功能，行政相对人认为该软件更新属于轻微软件更新，故软件发布版本是否可以不变？

答： 新增临床功能属于重大软件更新，软件发布版本亦需变更。若行政相对人制定的软件版本命名规则无法清晰区分重大和轻微软件更新，则遵循风险从高原则按重大软件更新处理。例如，软件版本命名规则为 X.Y.Z，其中 X 代表重大软件更新，Y 代表无法区分重大和轻微软件更新，Z 代表轻微软件更新，则软件发布版本命名为 X.Y。

24. 问：有源医疗器械的性能指标，进行检验时结果允差较大，不满足相关要求。可否依据检验报告数据直接修改该性能指标的标称值，以使检测结果的允差符合要求？

答： 产品的标称值是基于产品需求来确定的，允差是基于生产工艺和检验设备的偏差来综合考虑的，上述参数属于产品的设计特征，不能简单依据检验报告数据来进行文字性修改。

如果要修改标称值和允差，行政相对人应首先考虑变更前后是否涉及产品设计参数和质量管理体系的变化，如涉及上述变化，应修改相关参数，并提供变更后生产的样品重新进行检验。

25. 问：进口产品，原产国批准的主机和配合主机使用附件的适用范围不一致，在按系统整体申报时，是否可以综合主机与附件的适用范围作为在中国申请的适用范围？

答：如果产品在原产国是按照主机和配合使用附件分别注册，首先需按照《医疗器械注册单元划分指导原则》，确定二者是否可作为同一单元。

如果可以按照同一单元申报注册，则可以综合主机与附件在原产国上市时的适用范围进行申报。当二者适用范围不一致时应当选择二者共同包含的部分，并参考国内已批准同类产品的适用范围进行规范。但所申报适用范围不应超出原产国所批准的范围。

26. 问：超声软组织切割止血设备动物试验，如有多个代表型号的超声刀头，动物试验的动物头数、刀数应如何分配？

答：对于申报多个超声刀头的产品，可根据《超声软组织切割止血系统注册技术审查指导原则》"十、动物试验"项下"（四）动物试验要求"选择代表刀头进行试验。如果经确认有多个代表型号的超声刀头，不同型号的代表刀头应独立进行评价，刀数应独立进行计算。

对于急性动物试验，应当考虑多次切割对试验动物正常生理状态的影响，以确保后续每次切割的血管／组织都处于正常的生理状态。对于慢性动物试验，建议不要在同一只动物上对多个刀头进行试验，以避免出现异常情况但无法区分分析的问题。

27. 问：超声软组织切割止血设备在进行电磁兼容试验时，可否选择一个型号的刀头作为典型型号？

答： 普通的超声刀头（不包含换能器）仅传导声能，不传导电能，理论上对电磁兼容性能没有影响，但在进行电磁兼容检验时需配合刀头进行检验以完成产品必要的功能。

有些超声刀头为了识别一次性使用、收集刀头工作参数等功能，刀头内带有芯片（如 RFID），需要进行供电，对电磁兼容性能可能有影响，需考虑不同型号刀头的差异，选取典型型号进行检测。对于不带有芯片，不传导电信号、电能的超声刀头，可以选择一个型号刀头进行检测。

28. 问：微波消融设备的主机和消融针是否可单独申报注册？是否需限定配合使用情形？

答： 微波消融设备的主机和消融针可以作为同一注册单元整体申报，也可拆分成不同的注册单元单独申报。

微波消融设备的主机、线缆及消融针的匹配性要求很高，随意更换配合方式会影响微波输出的安全有效性，研发生产和使用必须与明确的主机或附件配合。

对于单独申报的微波消融设备的主机和消融针，均需明确配合使用产品的相关限定。单独申报的主机需在适用范围中明确配合已批准与本设备连用的消融针使用；单独申报的消融针需在适用范围中明确配合使用主机的规格型号和软件版本号。

29. 问：内窥镜动力设备包含哪些种类？各类产品的主要性能指标应当如何确定？

答： 内窥镜动力设备是指利用电源驱动动力装置为工具头提供机械动力，在内窥镜手术中对组织进行绞碎或切除的产品。内窥镜动力设备可根据工具头所实现的刨削、磨、钻等用途，分为不同的种类。例如，用于软组织刨削的设备、用于骨组织磨／钻的设备，以及同时包含以上两种功能的设备。

产品的主要性能指标应参照相应的国家标准、行业标准，并结合临床需求、自身产品的技术特点确定。其中，用于刨削的设备应符合行业标准 YY/T 0955《医用内窥镜内窥镜手术设备刨削器》的要求，用于其他用途（如磨、钻等）的设备可参照该标准同时结合产品特点确定相应的指标参数。

30. 问：高频超声集成手术设备，如果既可以单独输出高频或超声能量，又可以同时输出高频和超声能量，进行电磁兼容检验时应如何考虑测试模式？

答： 对于发射试验，按照 GB 4824《工业、科学和医疗设备射频骚扰特性限值和测量方法》规定，超声手术设备应为 1 组设备，高频手术设备为 2 组设备，但根据 GB 9706.4《医用电气设备第 2-2 部分：高频手术设备安全专用要求》/GB 9706.202《医用电气设备第 2-2 部分：高频手术设备及高频附件的基本安全和基本性能专用要求》相关要求，高频手术设备通电时并且高频输出未激励的空置状态下应符合第 1 组的限值要求。因此集成手术设备的发射试验应选择最不利模式（至少应包含最大超声输出模式）进行测试，按照1组A类进行试验。

对于抗扰度试验，应分别选择待机模式、超声输出模式、高频输出模式和双输出模式，在最不利情形下进行试验。

31. 问：有源手术设备包含多种手术器械，为针对不同科室需求提供不同种类及数量的手术器械，是否可将手术器械以"选配件"的形式申报注册？

答： 如果医疗器械的产品组成中某个部分是为了实现其预期用途和基本功能必不可少的，就不能作为"选配件"；如果手术器械预期就是可选配的，为了实现不同的功能选择不同型号使用，可以按照"选配件"的形式申报注册。单独购买或不购买某个或部分型号手术器械，并不影响产品整体使用的安全有效性。

无论手术器械是否以"选配件"形式申报注册，技术审评的要求都是一样的，都需要在产品的结构及组成中体现。

第二章

无源医疗器械产品技术共性问题

32. 问：软性角膜接触镜产品选择或变更初包装材料时应考虑哪些因素？

答： 软性角膜接触镜产品初包装材料中的游离物质有被溶液萃取的风险，可能影响接触镜的性能和安全性，因此在选择或变更初包装材料时应注意：

（1）对初包装材料的性能进行验证，包括理化性能和生物学评价（如可沥滤物分析、生物学试验等）。

（2）对初包装材料进行灭菌适用性研究及灭菌确认。

（3）建议按照 GB/T 11417.8《眼科光学接触镜 第 8 部分：有效期的确定》进行产品稳定性验证，建议包含镜片性能、包装完整性、无菌性能等，建议进行保存液性能研究。

（4）对初包装材料进行运输稳定性验证。

（5）如含有两种及两种以上初包装，应分别对不同初包装的终产品进行全性能检测及生物学评价，全性能包括全部设计验证的性能，以及技术要求中的全部性能指标。

（6）如采用从未在同类产品中应用的初包装材料，在稳定性试验中，建议对保存液中可能含有的沥滤物进行评价和验证。

33. 问：接触镜护理产品如宣称适用于硅水凝胶镜片，需提交哪些资料？有哪些注意事项？

答： 根据 YY 0719.5《眼科光学接触镜护理产品 第 5 部分：接触镜与接触镜护理产品物理相容性的测定》要求，应单独进行护理产品与硅水凝胶镜片的相容性试验。行政相对人应选择已上市的有代表性的硅水凝胶镜片进行研究并提交验证资料。产品技术要求中应明确检测时使用了硅水凝胶镜片，并提交行政相对人出具的自检报告或委托有资质的医疗器械检验机构出具的检验报告作为支持性资料。如未提交上述资料，适用范围中应明示不适用于硅水凝胶镜片。

34. 问：对于注射用交联透明质酸钠凝胶产品，若预灌封注射器为外购有注册证书的产品，是否需要在产品技术要求中制定相关性能要求？

答：鉴于预灌封注射器不仅作为器械的内包装容器，同时还具有注射的功能，因此无论其是否取得药品包装材料或医疗器械注册证书，均需从终产品的角度考虑在产品技术要求中，制定与之相关的可进行客观判定的功能性、安全性指标和检验方法，如推挤力、注射器外观、刻度、圆锥接头性能（对于非圆锥接头，需要求注射器与注射针的配合无泄漏）、有效容量（或装量）、器身密合性（活塞处无凝胶泄漏或用水进行测试）、活塞与外套的配合性（保持垂直时芯杆不因重力而移动）等，具体性能指标及试验方法可参照 GB 15810《一次性使用无菌注射器》或相关国家/行业标准。

35. 问：如宣称软性亲水接触镜为离子型或非离子型，应如何提交相关研究资料？

答：如行政相对人宣称软性亲水接触镜为离子型或非离子型，应依据 GB/T 11417.1《眼科光学接触镜 第1部分：词汇、分类和推荐的标识规范》中给出的离子型、非离子型的定义进行判定。首先需明确产品配方中各单体的性质，如离子型、非离子型等，其次计算离子型单体的含量（用摩尔分数表示），最后依据 GB/T 11417.1《眼科光学接触镜 第 1 部分：词汇、分类和推荐的标识规范》的相关要求做出结论，并在产品技术要求附录中明确软性亲水接触镜为离子型或非离子型。

36. 问：血管内导管产品在什么情况下应提供流量的研究资料，并且需要在产品技术要求中制定流量/流速要求？

答：（1）如果血管内导管产品的说明书/标签或其他资料中有标称流量，需提供流量的相关研究资料。

（2）对于向体内输注药液的导管，如中心静脉导管，应对流量/流速进行规定，同时在技术要求中制定流量/流速要求。

（3）因 YY 0285.1《血管内导管一次性使用无菌导管 第 1 部分：通用要求》附录 E 流量/流速检测方法中的灌注压力约为 10kPa，该标准中的流量要求不适用于标称流量的灌注压力大于 10kPa 的产品，对于灌注压力超过 10kPa 的产品，可不在产品技术要求中制定流量要求，但需在研究资料中提供相应验证资料。

37. 问：血管内造影导管产品在什么情况下应考虑动力注射要求，对于需要考虑动力注射要求的，申报资料中需注意哪些事项？

答：（1）对于采用高压注射装置注射的造影导管产品，需在技术要求和说明书（包括标签）中标注最大爆破压力信息，同时按照 YY 0285.1《血管内导管一次性使用无菌导管　第 1 部分：通用要求》在技术要求中对动力注射要求进行规定。

（2）对于采用环柄注射器注射造影剂的造影导管产品，可不制定动力注射要求，宜在说明书中明确以下警示：请勿使用高压注射装置注射造影剂。

（3）适用范围中包含血管造影功能的其他导管，宜参照以上要求。

38. 问：当使用行政相对人自己的已上市同类器械的生物学试验报告替代申报产品的生物学试验报告时，需要进行哪些考量？

答:（1）行政相对人需确认试验报告中的受试同类产品与申报产品在材料化学组成、各组成材料比例、产品物理结构、表面特性、生产工艺、灭菌方法、原材料供应商及技术规范、内包装材料（如适用，主要涉及液体类产品、湿态保存产品）等任何可能影响生物学风险的因素均完全一致，并提供相关声明。

（2）若受试品与申报产品在以上所列可能影响生物学风险的因素中存在不一致的情况，则需提供充分的理由和证据支持所提交的试验报告适用于申报产品，必要时补充相应的生物学评价资料，如可沥滤物分析及毒理学风险评定资料、相关生物学试验项目的补充试验等。

（3）同类产品的生物学试验报告仅用于替代申报产品试验报告，作为生物学评价的一部分，而不是替代申报产品整体的生物学评价报告。

39. 问：细胞毒性评价中定量评价和定性评价的选择原则是什么？优先推荐哪种评价方法？

答：细胞毒性的定量评价可以客观地对细胞数量、蛋白质总量、酶的释放、活体染料的释放、活体染料的还原或其他可测定的参数进行定量测定，不易受到试验者主观因素的影响，具有相对高的灵敏性且有明确的判定限，目前 MTT 定量法是国内普遍应用的方法。相对而言，细胞毒性的定性评价具有更多的评价者主观性，更适合筛选用途。

另外，实际测试中存在定性评价与定量评价的结果并不一致的情况（如受试样品浸提液存在使培养基吸光度出现较大变化的物质等）。因此推荐以定量评价法为基础，同时需要镜检细胞形态并报告结果，必要时辅以定性评价。

40. 问：动物源性医疗器械是否必须对病毒灭活工艺进行实验室验证以评价病毒灭活效果？

答：根据《动物源性医疗器械注册技术审查指导原则》，动物源性医疗器械注册申报时，提交的研究资料需包含对生产过程中病毒灭活和去除病毒和（或）传染性因子工艺过程的描述及有效性验证数据或相关资料。不同的动物来源、生产工艺以及适用范围的产品，风险各异。病毒灭活效果研究资料可以是通过实验室验证获取验证数据，或者从动物源材料供应商处获取验证数据。对于原材料应用比较成熟的产品，若其采用成熟的病毒灭活工艺且有相关的文献资料，也可以通过文献或历史数据对病毒灭活效果进行评价。若所提交的验证数据不是基于申报产品本身验证获得的数据，则需要进行适用性的分析论证。

41. 问：GB/T 16886.1《医疗器械生物学评价 第 1 部分：风险管理过程中的评价与试验》和《医疗器械生物学评价和审查指南》中都提及豁免生物学试验，手术器械类产品在什么情况下可以豁免生物学试验？

答：基于当前认知水平，若手术器械类产品中与患者直接或间接接触的材料仅由金属材料组成，经验证符合外科植入物用金属材料或外科器械用材料相关国家、行业及国际标准，以及相关产品标准中规定牌号，在提供材料化学成分验证资料（若论证生产工艺对材料化学成分不造成影响，可以原材料材质单的形式提交）的情况下可豁免生物学试验。

42. 问：注射用交联透明质酸钠凝胶产品，如含有外购已获注册证的注射针配件，配件应开展哪些性能研究？

答：对于注射用交联透明质酸钠凝胶产品，如含有外购已获注册证的注射针配件，应提交外购注射针的质控标准、测试报告和证明文件（如医疗器械注册证书等）。

（1）若所采购注射针为环氧乙烷（EO）灭菌，行政相对人需提供资料（如供应商检测报告或入厂检测报告等）证明注射针的 EO 残留风险已得到控制。鉴于 EO 残留风险在入厂时进行控制，且入厂后随放置时间风险降低，若生产环节不引入新的

EO 风险，可不在注射用交联透明质酸钠凝胶的产品技术要求中制定 EO 残留要求。

（2）若注射针未获得注册证书，需在研究资料中提供注射针的相关验证资料。行政相对人对外购配件的安全有效性负主体责任，因此应参照 GB 15811《一次性使用无菌注射针》在产品技术要求中制定注射针的性能要求和检测方法，并提供检验报告。

43. 问：含有输送系统或配件的无源血管植入器械，植入部件和输送系统或配件是否需要分别进行生物学评价？

答：对于含有输送系统或配件的无源血管植入性医疗器械，如预装在输送系统上的植入性支架、封堵器等，由于此类医疗器械中预计长期留置于人体的部件与其输送系统或配件在与人体接触性质和（或）接触时间方面存在明显不同，该类产品在注册时，宜对预期长期留置于人体的部件和输送系统或配件分别进行生物学评价，热原试验可合并进行。

44. 问：对于免于进行临床评价的疝修补补片，与《免于临床评价医疗器械目录》中已获境内注册产品进行机械性能对比时需要注意哪些方面？

答：对于免于进行临床评价的疝修补补片，当拉伸强度、拉伸伸长率、顶破强度符合临床使用标准时可不进行对比。若拉伸伸长率与临床接受标准存在出入则需与已获境内注册产品进行对比研究，论证其风险可接受。申报产品的单位面积重量、孔尺寸、孔隙率 / 网孔密度一般与《免于临床评价医疗器械目录》中已获境内注册产品相当；申报产品的撕裂强度（仅适用于裤形补片）、缝合强度、连接强度等，应不差于同类已上市产品。

45. 问：疝修补补片在制定拉伸强度和拉伸伸长率性能指标时应注意哪些方面？

答：（1）若材料设计、编织工艺等原因导致补片拉伸强度具有各向异性，应分别制定纵向、横向拉伸强度。

（2）建议制定人体生理条件可能受到的最大腹壁拉力下的拉伸伸长率。拉伸伸长率的接受标准应综合人体天然腹壁的伸长率情况及补片的实测数据制定。若材料设计、编织工艺等原因导致补片拉伸伸长率具有各向异性，应分别制定纵向、横向拉伸伸长率。

46. 问：增材制造口腔修复用激光选区熔化金属材料打印后为什么需要进行热处理，以及需提供哪些研究资料？

答：由于口腔修复用激光选区熔化金属材料在其打印成形过程中可能会产生热应力、组织应力、残余应力，容易导致终产品的翘曲变形与裂纹，使得终产品塑性较低，因此需要进行热处理。

一般热处理工艺包括回火、退火等。对热处理工艺的研究，一般需明确产品的热处理工艺方法及热处理工艺参数，对热处理方法的适宜性进行评估及验证，提供热处理工艺参数（如升温时间、保温温度、保温时间等）确定的依据，并论证热处理结果的临床可接受性。

47. 问：单髁膝关节假体性能研究至少应包括哪些内容?

答： 单髁膝关节假体一般为单间室膝关节假体，用于替代膝关节的内侧或外侧间室的股骨和胫骨关节面，通常包括股骨部件和胫骨部件，其中胫骨部件由胫骨衬垫和胫骨托组成。

行政相对人在设计研发该类产品时可参考 YY 0502《关节置换植入物膝关节假体》、YY/T 0919《无源外科植入物关节置换植入物膝关节置换植入物的专用要求》、YY/T 0924《外科植入物部分和全膝关节假体部件》系列标准等。产品的非临床研究至少应包括如下内容。

（1）关节面设计的相关研究资料。

（2）力学性能研究资料，一般包括股骨部件的疲劳性能、胫骨托的疲劳性能、关节磨损性能等。

（3）产品的生物学评价资料。

（4）产品的灭菌验证确认资料。

（5）产品货架有效期的验证资料。

48. 问：金属空心接骨螺钉的力学性能研究一般包括哪些内容?

答： 金属空心接骨螺钉的适用范围一般用于四肢骨折内固定，分为单独使用或配合金属接骨板使用两种情况，通常需要对其进行力学性能研究。

结合产品特点和预期用途，力学性能研究应至少评价螺钉的最大扭矩和断裂扭转角、轴向拔出性能、旋入扭矩和旋出扭矩性能，若螺钉还具备自攻能力，还应评价其自攻性能。其中对于旋入扭矩和旋出扭矩性能，行政相对人在产品设计过程中除了应考虑避免螺钉在旋入和旋出过程中断裂，还应确保临床医生方便轻松旋入和旋出，因此应注意螺钉的旋入扭矩和旋出扭矩不宜过大。

49. 问：自稳型椎间融合器的力学性能研究一般包括哪些内容？

答： 自稳型椎间融合器一般是由椎间融合器、金属板以及螺钉组成，因不需要额外配合脊柱内固定器械，常被称为自稳型椎间融合器，多用于颈椎部位的椎间融合术。

自稳型椎间融合器在开展力学性能评价时，既要考虑椎间融合器本身的性能，如压缩性能、压缩剪切性能、扭转性能、沉陷等，还应考虑用于替代脊柱内固定器械功能的金属板的性能，如压弯性能、扭转性能等，同时还应考虑金属板和椎间融合器的连接结构和系统结构的长期稳定性，螺钉的扭转性能和固定强度等。行政相对人可结合产品的结构特点，模拟临床使用方式，开展相关试验。

50. 问：胸腰椎后路内固定系统在进行系统性能试验时，试验样品的最差情形选择一般应考虑哪些内容？

答： 胸腰椎后路内固定系统性能试验一般包括系统压缩试

验、系统拉伸试验、系统扭转试验。系统性能试验最差情形样品在选择时需考虑产品的设计型式、尺寸规格、组配情况以及组件间的锁紧机制等因素，不同的性能试验的受力模式不同，对应最差情形的样品可能不同。通常系统动态疲劳试验中样品发生失效的情形除了椎弓根螺钉的螺纹根部断裂外，还可能发生连接棒失效，因此，确定试验样品的最差情形，应综合考虑连接棒的特点（如材质、规格、设计型式、表面处理方式）、组件间的锁紧方式及组配情况等对系统性能的影响。对于系统性能试验无法体现的组件风险，可通过组件试验进行评价，综合论证试验结果的临床可接受性。

51. 问：关节假体用涂层设计一般需考虑哪些方面？

答： 关节假体涂层主要是用于提高骨组织与非骨水泥固定关节假体的附着力，因此涂层的设计决定了预期的骨结合效果。

通常应明确的涂层参数至少包括涂层孔隙率、涂层厚度、涂层孔隙截距、涂层表面粗糙度（如适用）等。涂层参数设计的合理性可通过参考同类已上市产品的情况或已有的临床应用长期数据，作为支撑涂层设计可实现假体稳定固定的证据。对于采用新的涂层材料、新的涂层工艺或新的涂层参数设计的情形，可决策是否需要开展动物试验研究，以证明涂层的有效性。

52. 问：肩关节假体产品在注册申报时应注意哪些问题？

答： 肩关节假体一般包含关节盂部件和肱骨部件，常见的肩关节假体产品有正肩关节假体和反肩关节假体。若同一组件材料相同，不同组件作为整体配合使用的情况下，结构组成相似的正肩关节假体和反肩关节假体可以一同进行注册申报。

肩关节假体的性能评价应至少考虑各组件的力学强度、组件间的连接稳定性、关节面的磨损性能以及关节活动度等，若部件带涂层，还应考虑涂层的性能。

53. 问：可降解骨接合植入物的体外降解试验一般应考虑哪些方面？

答： 对于可降解骨接合植入物，为了保证其能为受损的骨组织提供坚强内固定，结合骨折愈合期，需评价其能够提供初始稳定性的能力。因此，一般需对可降解骨接合植入物进行降解性能的体外研究，研究内容应至少包括产品的降解速率、力学性能随降解过程中时间变化的情况、产品的降解产物以及产品的降解周期，产品降解性能试验的观察时间终点应考虑达到降解稳态或直至产品完全降解。

54. 问：髋关节假体中金属髋臼杯抗变形性能评价应注意哪些方面？

答： 金属髋臼杯抗变形性能评价的测试方法可参考 YY/T 0809.12《外科植入物部分和全髋关节假体 第 12 部分：髋臼杯形变测试方法》，按照该标准所述测试方法所得的初始直径的残差大于所得变形的 2%。此处所指 2% 并不是髋臼杯抗变形性能可接受的标准，而是说明产品发生塑性变形，此时应停止测试该试样，并选择新的试样重新测试。

行政相对人在评价髋臼杯抗变形性能时应提供测试结果可接受依据，应结合产品实际临床应用情况，考虑髋臼杯本身抗变形的能力和对髋臼内衬的影响。由于金属髋臼杯预期和髋臼内衬配合使用，测试时除考虑髋臼杯本身形变之外，还应考虑髋臼杯和内衬组配后的形变。

55. 问：开展椎间融合器力学性能研究时如何进行最差情形样品的选择？

答： 椎间融合器在开展力学性能研究时，通常应选择最差情形样品进行试验。用于颈椎的椎间融合器和用于胸腰椎的椎间融合器由于受力不同，应分别选择最差情形样品。应考虑不同型号规格融合器的植骨区尺寸、侧孔尺寸、倾角、长度、宽度和高度等因素对产品力学性能的影响。同时不同力学性能的受力情形不同，所选择的最差情形样品也可能不同，结合动、静态力学性能试验方法和加载方式，可采用有限元分析的方法分别确定颈椎和胸腰椎椎间融合器最差情形样品。

56. 问：在开展医疗器械产品各项性能研究时，是否需考虑产品批次对性能的影响？

答： 对于大多数医疗器械（非体外诊断试剂）而言，产品各项性能的稳定性和有效期通常取决于产品所用原材料和材料老化机理，如热老化、光老化等。在产品原材料性能、生产工艺和包装材料保持稳定的情况下，原则上批次间差异不应对产品各项性能稳定性和有效期产生影响。因此，一般情况下，在进行性能研究时，不需要考虑批次的问题。若产品具有特殊性，比如含有生物活性物质等，可以考虑批次间差异对产品性能的影响。

57. 问：无源医疗器械货架有效期研究中，若开展实时稳定性验证，应如何考虑验证温度？

答： 理论上产品实时稳定性研究的温度一般与储存温度相同，若某些产品有特殊规定，则优先执行相关规定，如 GB/T 11417.8《眼科光学接触镜 第 8 部分：有效期的确定》，该标准明确规定角膜接触镜产品稳定性研究采用的温度为 25℃。但对于常温保存的一般医疗器械，若无特殊规定，原则上不强制实时稳定性验证温度按照（25±2）℃进行，可依据产品特点提供相应的研究资料。对保存温度有特殊要求的医疗器械，应按照其规定温度进行验证研究。

58. 问：应如何评价同种异体医疗器械病毒灭活研究？

答： 同种异体医疗器械，即取材于人体组织制成的医疗器械，如同种异体骨、同种异体肌腱，需考虑产品病毒或传染性因子等生物安全性的风险，因此需对产品的病毒灭活工艺进行有效性验证研究。

对于一些常见的病毒灭活工艺，如有机溶剂、射线辐照、强酸强碱等，其过程和方法相对成熟，可参考的文献证据很多，对于原材料应用比较成熟的产品，行政相对人可通过文献或历史数据评价病毒灭活工艺效果，也可通过病毒灭活工艺验证试验评价病毒灭活效果。

59. 问：可吸收医疗器械产品在什么情形下可不开展体内代谢研究？

答： 可吸收医疗器械产品的原材料因为可以被人体吸收，其在体内的代谢可能存在安全风险，需关注其在人体内的代谢情况。然而对于大多数成熟材料，如透明质酸钠、动物胶原、壳聚糖、淀粉、聚乳酸等，相关研究文献资料较多，且其代谢路径相对固定，剂量、交联度和个体差异等对代谢路径影响较小，一般不会发生明显变化。因此，对于由上述成熟材料制备的产品，行政相对人可不提供产品的体内代谢研究资料，可通过提供已有的文献资料作为支持，或通过生物相容性评价等方式，验证产品的安全性。若产品采用新的可吸收材料，且缺乏对该材料体内代谢的相关研究资料，则需要进行该产品的体内代谢研究。

60. 问：产品技术要求中是否应规定产品材料性能指标？

答： 根据《医疗器械注册与备案管理办法》的要求，产品技术要求中的性能指标主要是指医疗器械成品的可进行客观判定的功能性、安全性指标，因此，一般产品材料性能不纳入产品技术要求的性能指标，包括但不限于金属类产品材料的化学成分、显微组织、内部质量等；高分子类产品材料的红外光谱等；陶瓷类产品材料的化学成分、杂质元素含量、导热系数、晶相含量等。对于确实与产品安全相关的材料表征信息，可在技术要求中以附录形式载明。

61. 问：不属于变更注册范围内的医疗器械产品说明书内容发生变化，应如何提交申请？

答：不属于变更注册范围内的医疗器械产品说明书内容发生变化，行政相对人可提交说明书更改告知申请。已注册医疗器械的说明书，除注册证及其附件载明事项之外的其他内容发生变化，不属于变更注册范围的，经审查同意后可进行更改。因此，不属于变更注册范围内的说明书内容发生变化，在提交说明书更改告知申请时，认为需提交相应证据的，行政相对人需将变化内容的支持性资料一并提交，审评人员需结合所提交的资料，综合审查是否允许更改。经审查认为不属于说明书更改告知范围的，需向行政相对人说明理由。

62. 问：骨科医疗器械若通过等同性测试证明与已上市产品等同，是否一定要选择性能最差情形的样品进行性能研究？

答：行政相对人提供的性能研究资料应始终围绕申报产品展开，考虑关键尺寸、结构设计等因素对产品性能的影响，对于不同的性能研究，分别选择相应最差情形的型号规格，进行相应试验，并评价试验结果的临床可接受性。在评价试验结果的临床可接受性时，可考虑通过等同性测试证明与已上市产品等同，即使申报产品与已上市产品具有相同的适用范围、适应证以及预期使用方式等（如：已有前代产品，申报产品与之相比仅在产品结构组成上存在一定差异），也应基于上述原则。

63. 问：增材制造口腔修复用激光选区熔化金属粉末与打印参数的匹配性应考虑哪些方面？

答： 增材制造用金属粉末与打印参数的匹配性主要涉及金属粉末的生产工艺及打印设备的关键工艺参数。关于金属粉末的生产工艺，应说明关键工艺原理及选择依据（如电极感应熔化气体雾化、等离子惰性气体雾化、真空感应熔化气体雾化、等离子旋转电极雾化等），明确关键工艺参数（如气体压力、流速和温度、气雾化喷嘴的内径和喷射角度、气雾化塔里的压力和氧含量、旋转电极雾化工艺的电流和转速等），并提交相关研究资料。关于与打印设备关键工艺参数的匹配性，应考虑激光功率、光斑直径、扫描速度、扫描间距、铺粉厚度、打印方向、气氛保护、支撑结构、成型室温度等工艺参数，并提交相关研究资料。

64. 问：骨科医疗器械若由符合 YY 0341.1《无源外科植入物骨接合与脊柱植入物 第1部分：骨接合植入物特殊要求》附录 B 中所述的临床使用证明可接受材料制成，是否可在提交注册申报资料时以豁免生物学评价的方式提交生物学评价资料？

答： 注册申报资料中的生物学评价资料是不能通过豁免生物学评价的方式提交的。行政相对人可通过等同性比较，证明申报产品与已上市产品具有相同的生物相容性，从而确定申报产品的生物学试验的减化或免除。对于符合 YY 0341.1《无源外科植入物骨接合与脊柱植入物 第 1 部分：骨接合植入物特殊要求》附录 B 中所述的材料，仍需通过等同性比较的方式进行生物学评价，同时考虑原材料的结构形态、产品结构特征以及生产过程等方面与已上市产品的差异对产品生物相容性的影响。以生产过程为例，产品的生产加工过程通常会引入新的有害物质（如灭菌剂、加工助剂、脱模剂等残留物），因此应评价申报产品的生产加工过程（加工过程、灭菌过程、包装等）是否引入新的、相同的风险，若经评价，申报产品没有引入新的生物学风险，则可豁免生物学试验。

65. 问：可吸收骨植入产品降解性能应如何评价？

答： 可吸收骨植入产品一般应开展产品降解性能研究，在研究过程中应关注与骨生长的匹配情况。产品设计应保证产品在降解初期能维持一段时间的初始稳定性。对于需提供一定力学强度的产品，如可吸收界面螺钉，产品在降解初期应具备一定的力学强度。因此在开展产品降解性能研究时，应关注产品的降解速率，结合临床骨生长所需的时间，评价产品在降解过程中的力学性能变化，确保产品降解初期的力学强度能够满足临床需要，同时保证产品的降解速率匹配骨生长的速率。建议行政相对人结合产品材料特性、结构设计及临床预期用途进行综合评价，可通过文献研究、同品种产品比对等方式提供相关支持性依据。

66. 问：常规超高分子量聚乙烯单髁膝关节假体的衬垫厚度是否必须至少达到 6mm?

答：原则上常规超高分子量聚乙烯材料制成的单髁膝关节衬垫在配合胫骨托部件使用时，其承受负载部位的厚度应至少达到 6mm。若产品设计不能满足该厚度，应提供产品设计依据和合理理由，并证明该设计能够保证产品满足临床安全有效性，提供相应的支持性依据。若与已上市同品种产品进行对比，应提供申报产品与已上市同品种产品在结构设计、关键尺寸及力学性能等方面的对比，并结合已上市同品种产品的临床应用情况，进行综合评价，并且可通过检索同品种产品的临床文献数据、不良事件数据等方式提供相关支持性证据。

67. 问：对于常规超高分子量聚乙烯材料骨科植入产品，YY/T 0772.3《外科植入物 超高分子量聚乙烯 第 3 部分：加速老化方法》中的加速老化试验和产品稳定性研究中的加速老化试验能否相互替代？

答：不能。对于常规超高分子量聚乙烯骨科植入产品，行政相对人应在研究资料中参照 YY/T 0772.3《外科植入物 超高分子量聚乙烯 第 3 部分：加速老化方法》、YY/T 0772.4《外科植入物 超高分子量聚乙烯 第 4 部分：氧化指数测试方法》、YY/T 0772.5《外科植入物 超高分子量聚乙烯 第 5 部分：形态评价方法》标准中的方法对常规超高分子量聚乙烯材料的稳定性（如：老化前后的氧化指数、力学性能）及形态学进行评价，该方法不能模拟出试验条件与产品实时储存老化之间的关系，因此并不能等同于产品稳定性研究。产品稳定性研究中的加速老化试验的试验条件是通过假设材料变质所涉及的化学反应遵循阿列纽斯函数，可推断产品在正常储存条件下材料老化情况。因此，产品的稳定性（包括货架有效期）研究应参照《无源植入性医疗器械稳定性研究指导原则》，提交产品实时稳定性或加速稳定性研究资料。

68. 问：一次性使用注射笔用针头产品，针头与注射笔的适配性需要验证哪些项目？

答： 行政相对人应提供申报产品与注射笔配合使用的相关验证资料。性能指标一般包括针座装配性能、针头剂量准确度、针座拆卸扭矩等。通过施加规定的扭矩将针头连接到注射笔，通过剂量精度测试确认临床相关的流体通路的完整性，测量并记录针座的拆卸扭矩。此外，提交申报产品与所宣称配合使用的注射笔功能适配性验证资料，对于所验证产品数量应提供合理性说明，明确置信度、可靠性等参数。

69. 问：血液透析器产品的清除率试验条件应如何设计？

答： 清除率是透析器的主要功能参数，也是评价透析器质量的关键指标。应明确清除率的试验条件，清除率试验应覆盖行政相对人所规定的血液流速和透析液流速范围。根据YY 0053《血液透析及相关治疗血液透析器、血液透析滤过器、血液滤过器和血液浓缩器》规定，透析器产品的清除率试验中，血液和透析液流速应覆盖行政相对人规定的范围。试验中透析液流速一般选择最低和最高点，同时分别对应说明书中规定的全部血液流速。

70. 问：灌流器产品需要控制哪些可沥滤物？

答：首先，行政相对人应严格限制原材料、生产工艺等过程中相关高风险物质的使用，以确保其残留满足预期使用条件下的安全性要求，并确保批次间稳定，或者进行相关高风险物质的替代研究。其次，应对各环节可能引入到终产品的可沥滤物进行充分的风险评估，如单体、溶剂、催化剂、交联剂等，还有一些原材料制备过程中可能出现的副产物，如二乙烯苯制备时可能出现的副产物萘等。

71. 问：高通量血液透析器产品的清除率检测中 β_2 微球蛋白清除率试验条件，是否可以只设置一个血液流速，不覆盖所有血液流速范围？

答：清除率是透析器的主要功能参数，也是评价透析器质量的关键指标。常用尿素、肌酐、磷酸盐、维生素 B_{12} 的清除率作为评价透析器滤除性能的指标，对于高通量透析器还应提供 β_2 微球蛋白的清除率性能测试或临床评估资料。根据 YY 0053《血液透析及相关治疗血液透析器、血液透析滤过器、血液滤过器和血液浓缩器》规定，高通量血液透析器应在临床常用血液流速下，可以选择单一血液流速，评价 β_2 微球蛋白清除率。

72. 问：如何理解《免于临床评价医疗器械目录》中输注产品不予豁免的情况？

答：《免于临床评价医疗器械目录》中输注产品规定了"豁免情况不包括新材料、新作用机理、新功能的产品"。新材料、新作用机理、新功能仅指在国内已上市同类输注器具中没有使用过的材料、作用机理和功能。

（1）新材料方面，如输液器管路聚氯乙烯（PVC）原材料中的偏苯三酸三辛酯（TOTM）增塑剂，已经在同类上市产品中使用。采用 TOTM 增塑剂 PVC 原材料制造的输液器，不属于新材料范畴，可以免除该产品的临床评价。

（2）新作用机理方面，如输液器采用浮体式或膜式止液组件，而同样组件已经在同类上市产品中使用，申报注册时其作用机理不属于新作用机理的范畴，可以免除该产品的临床评价。

（3）新功能方面，如输液针具有防针刺功能，而该功能已经在同类上市产品中使用，申报注册时不属于新功能范畴，可以免除该产品的临床评价。

73. 问：应用纳米材料的医疗器械，应如何对其进行风险评估？

答： 应用纳米材料的医疗器械需符合 GB/T 16886.1《医疗器械生物学评价 第 1 部分：风险管理过程中的评价与试验》、YY/T 0316《医疗器械 风险管理对医疗器械的应用》和《医疗器械产品受益 – 风险评估注册技术审查指导原则》等文件中规定的风险因素，主要包括纳米材料从器械释放的可能性、暴露剂量、暴露途径、接触部位和暴露时间。

风险评估最重要的因素是纳米材料从医疗器械中释放的可能性。风险评估应分阶段、有步骤进行，考虑暴露评估（纳米材料释放）、纳米材料分布及持续存留和环境转化、危害识别，并最终根据产品的适用范围是否给患者带来足够的受益来综合考虑产品风险。

74. 问：应用纳米材料的医疗器械，应如何考虑安全性问题？

答：由于纳米材料的比表面积等因素不同，纳米材料表现出不同的理化性质，因此，生物体暴露于纳米材料之后，可能表现出与常规材料不同的生物学反应。行政相对人应针对医疗器械的结构特征、预期用途、与人体的接触途径、所含纳米材料的种类和形态等因素，通过设计一系列试验来确认测试系统的适用性，从而建立起适合所申报产品特点的生物学评价方案，从而保证产品的安全性。

GB/T 16886《医疗器械生物学评价》系列标准的生物学评价体系总体适用于纳米材料，但具体到某一应用纳米材料的医疗器械，其试验方法、样品制备、细胞系/动物品系选择、观察终点、结果分析等均可能与常规材料不同，需结合产品特点进行评价。

75. 问：一次性使用高压造影注射器及附件的产品性能指标包括哪些内容？

答： 产品的性能指标包括但不限于以下几点：① 外观；② 保护套和保护帽不应自然脱落且易于拆除；③ 与外界隔离（如适用）；④ 鲁尔圆锥接头符合 GB/T 1962《注射器、注射针及其他医疗器械 6%（鲁尔）圆锥接头》系列标准的要求；⑤ 微粒污染；⑥ 造影注射器（润滑剂、透明度、刻度线与标志、圆锥接头、密合性）；⑦ 穿刺式吸药器瓶塞穿刺器及进气器件符合 YY 0804《药液转移器 要求和试验方法》要求；⑧ 管式吸药器与注射器相适且壁厚不小于 0.5mm；⑨ 连接管路（尺寸、连接牢固性、密合性、单向阀）；⑩ 可萃取金属含量；⑪ 酸碱度；⑫ 易氧化物；⑬ 环氧乙烷残留（如适用）；⑭ 无菌；⑮ 细菌内毒素。行政相对人还应提交申报产品与高压造影注射设备的适配性研究资料。

76. 问：一次性使用硬膜外麻醉导管注册申报时生物学评价是否必须进行亚慢性毒性、遗传毒性和植入评价？

答： 根据 GB/T 16886.1《医疗器械生物学评价 第 1 部分：风险管理过程中的评价与试验》标准要求，如硬膜外麻醉导管产品与人体持续接触时间小于 30 天，则无需进行亚慢性毒性、遗传毒性和植入评价；而用于晚期癌症硬膜镇痛的产品，如用于晚期癌症硬膜镇痛的硬膜外麻醉导管，其与人体持续接触大于 30 天，则需要进行亚慢性毒性、遗传毒性和植入评价。

77. 问：如何验证一次性使用内窥镜注射针与内窥镜的配合性能？

答： 行政相对人应明确各型号内镜注射针推荐配合使用内窥镜钳道的尺寸。提供配合性能的研究资料，包括产品模拟临床使用时，内镜注射针配合使用内窥镜（或内镜模拟钳道，模拟钳道应提供设计依据信息以证明其符合临床实际）能自由进出，无明显阻力、卡塞、扭曲现象，各部件操作灵活并符合使用要求，多次出针及收针均正常顺畅，连接部位无断裂、脱离等不良现象。

78. 问：用于血液透析机内部管路消毒的柠檬酸消毒液，其性能研究至少包括哪些内容？

答： 用于血液透析机内部管路加热消毒的柠檬酸消毒液的主要成分为柠檬酸，一般还可以包含乳酸和苹果酸。

该类产品的性能研究至少包括：外观、酸碱度、装量、产品主要有效成分（柠檬酸等含量）、有效期、对金属腐蚀性、杀灭微生物指标等。如产品主要有效成分包含特殊物质，或其他非同类已上市产品功能的，应规定相应物质成分、含量和使用性能。

79. 问：凡士林纱布产品对原材料有哪些要求？

答： 凡士林纱布一般用于烧伤、烫伤、皮肤移植的供皮区和植皮区等的创面保护和填塞，以及需要引流的渗液型伤口。YY/T 1293.1《接触性创面敷料 第1部分：凡士林纱布》规定了该类产品的性能要求。凡士林应符合《中华人民共和国药典》要求，进口产品可参考美国药典或欧洲药典等要求。脱脂棉纱布或脱脂棉粘胶混纺纱布建议参考 YY 0331《脱脂棉纱布、脱脂棉粘胶混纺纱布的性能要求和试验方法》要求。

80. 问：针对肾功能衰竭患者的血液净化产品生物学评价应如何考虑？

答： 参照 GB/T 16886《医疗器械生物学评价》系列标准，总体生物学评价应考虑以下方面：

（1）制造所用材料；

（2）预期的添加剂、工艺污染物和残留物；

（3）可沥滤物质；

（4）降解产物（如适用）；

（5）其他组件及其在最终产品中的相互作用；

（6）最终产品的性能与特点；

（7）最终产品的物理特性，包括但不限于：多孔性、颗粒大小、性状和表面形态；

（8）根据血液净化产品临床预期用途，产品的生物学评价应考虑累计作用时间，按照外部接入器械与循环血液持久接触要求进行。如果产品采用全新材料，或可能含有致癌性、致突变性和（或）生殖毒性物质，还建议在风险评定中考虑相关终点。

第三章

体外诊断试剂产品技术共性问题

81. 问：什么是体外诊断试剂的检测系统？如果体外诊断试剂注册过程中，不包含检测系统的全部组分，是否需要将该产品检测系统予以明确？

答：体外诊断试剂的检测系统是指由样本处理用产品、检测试剂、校准品、质控品、检测设备等构成的，可完成样本从处理到最终结果报告所有阶段的组合。整个检测系统经过充分的安全有效性评价并获得批准。

体外诊断试剂在产品注册过程中，可能未包含完成检测的所有其他产品，此时需要将配套的产品在说明书中予以明确，确保检测过程按照所有配套产品组成的检测系统进行。例如，对于不包括提取试剂的核酸检测试剂，在性能评估和临床评价过程中，均需采用说明书声称的配套提取试剂。

同样，申报资料中如果涉及对比试剂，亦要按其批准的检测系统进行操作。例如，采用对比试剂说明书声称的配套提取试剂提取核酸，并进行后续检测，其获得的检测结果可以作为评价考核试剂的依据。

82. 问：基于二代测序技术的体外诊断试剂盒，是否应将预建库试剂包含于试剂盒的组成中进行注册申报？

答：预建库试剂一般包含末端修复、接头连接和扩增等预文库制备相关组分，用于完成对基因测序文库的通用处理，后续需采用试剂盒中其他组分进行文库的特异性识别或富集。考虑到预文库制备步骤在基于二代测序技术的检测中为关键步骤，预建库试剂的质量是否稳定，直接影响到检测结果的准确性。因此，行政相对人应将预建库试剂包含于试剂盒的组成中进行注册申报，以便控制产品的稳定性。值得注意的是，医疗器械分类目录中目前已有分类界定的（预）建库试剂，管理类别均为三类，所以，不可将预建库试剂单独拆分进行备案。

83. 问：申请体外诊断设备变更注册时，什么情况下需要补充网络安全的检验报告？

答：依据《医疗器械网络安全注册技术审查指导原则》，行政相对人需在产品技术要求性能指标中明确数据接口、用户访问控制的要求。该指导原则发布之前批准的产品如未体现以上指标，建议提交变更注册申请，补充完善相关指标。申请其他变更事项时，若涉及网络安全内容，行政相对人有必要在产品技术要求中补充网络安全的性能指标。以上两种情况均需提供补充项目的检验报告，同时需提交网络安全描述文档，作为变更的支持性资料。

84. 问：体外诊断试剂包装规格的变更申请，需要提交什么资料？

答：体外诊断试剂包装规格发生变化，应详细描述变更前后包装规格的差异，根据具体差异，识别所有相关的潜在风险，并针对这些风险因素进行分析和验证。例如：① 变更前后包装规格的反应形式（如毒品类检测产品）、反应膜条大小（如 PCR 扩增杂交法产品）存在差异，应提交变更后包装规格的分析性能评估资料；②变更前后包装规格的装量或容器发生显著变化，导致其蒸发、损耗等风险增加，应考虑产品的货架有效期、使用稳定性及校准频率等是否发生变化。

85. 问：体外诊断试剂变更注册申请中"（二）概述：详细描述本次变更情况、变更的具体原因及目的"应包含什么内容？

答： 在进行变更注册申请时，要详述变更的原因及目的，说明变更的根本原因。对于性能声称有所提升的，应详述如何通过优化实现性能的提升。对于进口产品的说明书变更原因，描述为"根据原文说明书进行更新"的同时，还需说明原文说明书发生变化的原因。建议详尽描述变更情况，列明产品的所有设计变更内容，并声明其余均未发生变化。

86. 问：降钙素原检测试剂什么情况下可以免于进行临床试验？

答： 降钙素原检测试剂用于体外定量测定人血清或血浆样本中的降钙素原。降钙素原检测试剂已列入《免于临床试验体外诊断试剂目录》，目录中预期用途为用于检测人体样本中的降钙素原（PCT）的含量，临床上主要用于细菌感染性疾病的辅助诊断。行政相对人如申报降钙素原检测试剂用于细菌感染性疾病的辅助诊断用途，包括对不同程度细菌感染的辅助诊断，可按照免临床的评价路径进行申报。行政相对人如申报降钙素原检测试剂的其他预期用途，则不属于《免于临床试验体外诊断试剂目录》范围，需开展临床试验以确认其声称的预期用途。

87. 问：基于酶联免疫法的体外诊断试剂，是否可通过变更注册将反应模式由"两步法"变为"一步法"？

答： 酶联免疫检验方法根据反应模式分为"一步法"和"两步法"。"一步法"是将待测样本和酶标记抗体同时加入到反应孔中进行反应，"两步法"则是先将样本加入到反应孔中，待该步骤反应结束后再加入酶标记抗体。两种方法的实验步骤不同，前者缩短了反应时间，但可能导致产品性能降低。所以，不建议通过变更注册将"两步法"变为"一步法"。

88. 问：医疗器械说明书发生变化该怎么办？

答： 根据《医疗器械说明书和标签管理规定》第十六条规定："已注册的医疗器械发生注册变更的，申请人应当在取得变更文件后，依据变更文件自行修改说明书和标签。"

已注册医疗器械的说明书，除注册证及其附件载明事项之外的其他内容发生变化，不属于变更注册范围的，应当向医疗器械注册的审批部门书面告知，并提交说明书更改情况对比说明等相关文件。

89. 问：定性检测试剂的干扰试验结果是否可仅采用阴/阳性表示？

答： 干扰试验一般采用配对比对的方式，比较含有高浓度干扰物质的样本与不含或含正常浓度干扰物质样本（对照）检测结果的差异。对于结果无量值数据的定性检测试剂，干扰试验结果可仅采用阴/阳性表示，但是应注意研究用样本需包含弱阳性水平；对基于量值数据（如 OD 值、Ct 值或计数结果等）进行阈值判断的定性检测试剂，建议对量值数据进行差异分析，而不是仅采用阴/阳性表示干扰试验的结果。

90. 问：关于调整《6840 体外诊断试剂分类子目录（2013 版）》部分内容的公告对哪些试剂的管理类别进行了调整？

答：国家药监局于 2020 年 10 月发布了关于调整《6840 体外诊断试剂分类子目录（2013 版）》部分内容的公告（2020 年第 112 号），对部分用于治疗监测的肿瘤标志物相关试剂管理类别调整为第 II 类，《6840 体外诊断试剂分类子目录（2013 版）》中用于辅助诊断用途的肿瘤标志物相关试剂，未进行类别调整，继续按照第 III 类管理。

91. 问：应如何规范新型冠状病毒抗原检测试剂说明书格式？

答：新型冠状病毒抗原检测试剂的说明书格式除了需要符合《体外诊断试剂说明书编写指导原则》，还需要根据《新型冠状病毒（2019-nCoV）抗原检测试剂注册审查指导原则》的附件《新型冠状病毒（2019-nCoV）抗原检测试剂盒（××××法）说明书》模板，结合申报产品情况进行规范，例如预期用途、采样步骤、采样注意事项、检验方法注意事项、局限性等。对于模板中斜体、粗体、黑体、下划线内容也应与其保持格式一致。

92. 问：聚合酶链反应（PCR）检测设备的临床项目分析性能研究中，评价用的试剂是否必须为已上市试剂？

答：PCR 检测设备的临床项目分析性能研究，其目的是为了评价设备和试剂整个检测系统在代表性临床项目上的分析性能，评价用的配套试剂应为成熟可靠的试剂。一般应当采用已上市试剂进行研究。常规的 PCR 检测设备为开放平台，可以配套多种已上市试剂。对于特殊的 PCR 检测设备，如确无配套的已上市试剂，可以采用未上市但已定型的试剂进行研究。

93. 问：体外诊断试剂稳定性研究，对于储存条件有什么要求？

答：体外诊断试剂稳定性是在制造商规定界限内保持其性能特性的能力。在进行试剂稳定性研究时，应充分考虑可能影响试剂性能或效果的变量，考虑环境因素的变化，包括最不利情形。研究过程中试剂应储存在制造商规定的条件下，该条件根据测试用设备的能力或试剂的预期储存条件来设定，应能充分验证最不利条件下的试剂稳定性。研究结果应能证明申报试剂在声称的储存条件和时间内能够满足稳定性要求。建议行政相对人在研究资料和稳定性声称中明确储存条件的具体范围（例如"2~8℃条件下保存"），不建议采用"冷藏""冷冻""室温"等不确定字样描述储存温度。

94. 问：体外诊断试剂产品技术要求的性能指标中是否必须纳入"稳定性"指标？

答： 依据《医疗器械产品技术要求编写指导原则》"四、性能指标要求"，"医疗器械货架有效期"属于"不建议在技术要求性能指标中规定的研究性及评价性内容"。此建议也适用于体外诊断试剂的产品技术要求，"稳定性"可不纳入体外诊断试剂产品技术要求的性能指标中。

95. 问：如何选择细菌耐药基因检测试剂的临床对比方法？

答： 细菌耐药基因检测试剂是指通过检测目标细菌特定耐药基因对其耐药情况进行判定的检测试剂。对此类试剂进行临床研究时，应首先选择临床耐药表型的结果作为临床参考标准进行对比研究，将基因检测结果与临床耐药检测结果进行比较，从而获得基因检测试剂对耐药菌检测的灵敏度和特异度。试剂对临床样本相关基因的检测性能可通过与基因测序或同类已上市产品比较研究的方式进行确认。

对于被测耐药基因位点在临床应用中较为公认且同类产品已上市多年的检测试剂，临床试验可以与同类已上市产品比较研究的方式为主，部分样本采用与耐药表型比对的方式进一步确认。如有适用的产品类指导原则，应参考相关指导原则要求。

96. 问：体外诊断试剂临床试验中是否可以进行阳性判断值 / 参考区间的调整？

答： 一般情况下，体外诊断试剂的阳性判断值 / 参考区间建立和验证工作完成后，才会进行临床试验。在临床试验中根据已经经过充分验证的阳性判断值 / 参考区间进行检测结果的判读。如果临床试验中依据临床参考标准认为试验体外诊断试剂的阳性判断值 / 参考区间的设定不合理且需要调整，调整后数据则将作为阳性判断值 / 参考区间研究数据，而非确认产品临床性能的临床研究数据。调整后需要重新入组临床病例进行临床试验。

97. 问：体外诊断试剂临床试验过程中针对试验体外诊断试剂与对比试剂检测结果不一致的样本，复测结果是否能够纳入最终的一致性统计？

答： 体外诊断试剂临床试验过程中，为了控制试验偏倚，针对试验体外诊断试剂与对比试剂的一致性统计分析，应采用样本揭盲前的检测结果。针对不一致样本，如按照临床试验方案规定进行了复测，复测结果为试验揭盲后再次检测的结果，纳入统计分析会引入偏倚，因此，不建议将此部分结果纳入总体统计分析。但试验体外诊断试剂复测结果可结合第三方复核试剂检测结果及该样本对应病例的临床诊断信息，进一步分析试验体外诊断试剂与对比试剂检测结果不一致的原因。

98. 问：体外诊断试剂临床试验中对产品说明书的关注点有哪些？

答： 体外诊断试剂临床试验设计和执行过程中，应特别关注临床试验过程中的操作细节与相关产品说明书的一致性，其中涉及的说明书包括试验体外诊断试剂说明书、对比试剂说明书以及复核试剂说明书。

无论是试验体外诊断试剂还是对比试剂、复核试剂，临床试验中应特别关注的说明书内容包括预期用途、适用样本类型、样本抗凝剂、样本保存及处理要求、样本处理用配套试剂（如核酸提取试剂）及其他配套试剂、适用机型、试验方法、结果判读标准、局限性等。

临床试验设计过程中应根据相关说明书规定，制定详细的标准操作规程，确保临床试验执行过程中试验体外诊断试剂、对比试剂、复核试剂的检测严格按照说明书要求操作，临床试验检测过程及结果应能支持拟申报产品说明书的声称内容。

99. 问：体外诊断试剂注册申报提交伦理文件与临床试验方案应注意哪些事项？

答： 体外诊断试剂临床试验资料中应提交临床试验执行的方案及与之对应的同意开展临床试验的伦理委员会书面意见。

由于临床试验方案的变更，可能存在多个版本号，提交申报资料时应注意以下原则：

如临床试验方案的变更发生在临床试验正式开展之前，应提交临床试验最终执行的版本号的临床试验方案，以及该版本号方案对应的伦理委员会书面意见。

如临床试验已经开始，执行过程中发生方案变更，需提交最终版本的临床试验方案和知情同意书，历次变更的伦理委员会意见。最终版本的临床试验方案，应详细列明历次变更情况；如未列明，则需提交历次变更的临床试验方案。申请人应明确说明方案变更的原因及其对已开展的临床试验的影响。

应当注意，临床试验之前应充分研究方案的科学性、合理性、可行性及合规性，制定方案并严格执行；临床试验过程中非必要原因不得随意对方案进行更改。

100. 问：体外诊断试剂临床试验中对样本使用的抗凝剂有何要求？

体外诊断试剂的检测样本涉及不同抗凝剂时，应在临床前研究阶段对不同抗凝剂进行研究，验证抗凝剂的适用性及其对检测的影响。

一般情况下，如经前期研究认为说明书声称可用的抗凝剂对样本检测不存在差异性影响，则临床试验过程中无需分组纳入使用不同抗凝剂的样本，所有适用的抗凝剂均可在临床试验样本中使用；特殊情形下当不同抗凝剂对检测结果有显著影响，导致临床检测结果的判定有不同参考值等情形，则临床试验中应分别进行样本收集和研究。临床试验方案和报告中应明确说明样本类型及样本使用的抗凝剂。

101. 问：进行体外诊断试剂临床试验时，关于样本应注意的问题有哪些？

答： 样本是体外诊断试剂临床试验中非常关键的要素，临床试验中应关注样本采集、样本保存条件、样本保存时间、样本处理方式等，应满足试验体外诊断试剂临床前研究确定的要求，严格按照说明书对样本进行全流程管理，应同步关注试验体外诊断试剂和对比试剂说明书要求。

例如，核酸检测试剂临床试验时应注意：

（1）应采用临床原始样本进行临床试验，提取的 DNA 或 RNA 核酸不视为原始样本；

（2）应采用试验体外诊断试剂和对比试剂各自产品说明书配套的核酸提取 / 纯化试剂、样本保存液（如适用）进行临床试验；

（3）如产品说明书对提取的核酸纯度和浓度有要求，应满足各自产品说明书的相关要求；

（4）样本保存条件、保存时间应符合要求；

（5）样本采样管、保存液、灭活等操作应符合说明书要求。

102. 问：抗肿瘤药物的非原研伴随诊断试剂研发时基因突变位点的覆盖范围应考虑哪些因素？

答： 对于抗肿瘤药物的非原研伴随诊断基因突变检测试剂，在产品研发时应充分考虑产品设计中基因的选择和位点的覆盖范围。如该基因针对相同的伴随诊断用途（如相同的伴随药物）

已知有多种突变位点，则后续产品设计时应结合产品风险受益分析充分考虑突变位点的覆盖程度，不应为了产品评价的易操作性随意缩小位点的检测范围。例如 *KRAS* 基因突变用于肿瘤伴随诊断时，因为其为负向伴随诊断基因检测且与药物不良反应相关，突变位点覆盖不足可能增加患者风险，产品设计时应充分参考原研产品或药物临床试验的基因覆盖情况。

103. 问：使用体外诊断试剂境外临床试验数据注册申报时应注意哪些问题？

答： 使用境外临床试验数据作为临床证据在我国进行注册申报时，行政相对人应提交境外临床试验机构的伦理意见、临床试验方案和临床试验报告。伦理意见、临床试验方案和临床试验报告的形式、内容与签字等应满足境外临床试验所在国家（地区）临床试验质量管理的相关要求。此外，行政相对人还应提交境内外临床试验相关因素的差异分析报告，详细说明体外诊断试剂在进行境外临床试验时相关因素与境内存在的差异以及针对差异的处理措施。必要时，还应提交境外临床试验所在国家（地区）有关临床试验质量管理的相关法律、法规、规范或标准等文件。

行政相对人应提供完整的境外临床试验数据，不得筛选，境外临床试验报告应包含对完整临床试验数据的分析及结论。

104. 问：体外诊断试剂临床试验设计中应如何制定受试者入组和排除标准？

答： 体外诊断试剂临床试验中应根据产品预期用途中的适用人群和适应证设定合理的受试者入组和排除标准。应当注意：临床试验受试者应来自产品预期用途所声称的适用人群（目标人群）和适应证，如具有某种症状、体征、生理、病理状态或某种流行病学背景等情况的人。非目标人群入组可能引入受试者选择偏倚，导致临床试验结果不能反映产品的真实情况。

例如，用于某种疾病辅助诊断的体外诊断试剂，临床试验中不应随意入组大量无症状健康受试者；乙肝、丙肝、艾滋、梅毒等相关检测试剂的临床试验不应大量入组无相关症状、体征的术前筛查患者。上述入组标准均可能导致产品临床特异性评价偏离产品的真实性能。

105. 问：伴随诊断试剂通过桥接试验路径作为伴随诊断临床证据时应注意哪些问题？

答： 桥接试验是使用试验体外诊断试剂对已经完成的关键性药物临床试验过程中入组患者的剩余样本进行检测，进而评估试验体外诊断试剂所确定的受试者的治疗效果。

伴随诊断试剂通过桥接试验路径作为伴随诊断临床证据时应注意：

（1）首先应确认支持药物境内上市的关键性药物临床试验，桥接试验应纳入该关键性临床试验中的所有入组病例的剩余样本，如因某些客观因素导致无法入组的，如样本量不够、缺少知情同意等，允许一部分脱落，但脱落的数量不应影响整体的评价；

（2）如药物临床试验为国际多中心临床试验，则桥接试验不仅要纳入境内病例的剩余样本，同时要纳入所有境外病例的剩余样本；

（3）如药物临床试验为富集性试验设计，入组病例可能仅为标志物检测阳性的病例，或者药物临床试验中的阴性病例不足，则桥接试验除纳入药物临床试验的入组病例的剩余样本外，还需要入组部分非药物临床试验的病例样本，用于评估试验体外诊断试剂与原研伴随诊断试剂或临床试验检测（CTA）的临床性能。该部分补充病例的入排标准应严格设定，应为试验体外诊断试剂的适用人群。针对额外入组的这部分阴性样本，需要采用试验体外诊断试剂和原研伴随诊断试剂或CTA同步进行检测。

106. 问：体外诊断试剂临床试验数据库的递交应注意哪些问题？

答：按照《关于公布体外诊断试剂注册申报资料要求和批准证明文件格式的公告》的要求，自2022年1月1日起，所有通过临床试验路径进行临床评价的体外诊断试剂均应提交临床试验数据库。行政相对人应按照《体外诊断试剂临床试验数据递交要求注册审查指导原则》的要求正确递交临床试验数据库。临床试验数据库应包括原始数据库、分析数据库、说明性文件、程序代码（如有）。

原始数据库指临床试验按照方案的要求入组的所有病例及样本信息，包括试验过程中进行了剔除的病例，同时应备注剔除原因；行政相对人应提供各机构的原始数据集以及汇总的原始数据集。

分析数据库指便于统计分析使用原始数据集形成的数据库，用于产生临床试验报告中的统计结果，应包括用于统计分析的相应的病例及样本信息；通常由多个不同的数据集组成，其中的数据集形成应与临床试验报告中的统计结果相对应。

说明性文件至少应包括数据说明文件以及统计分析说明文件。根据采用不同的统计分析工具，应在统计分析说明文件中阐明统计分析过程以便易于审评过程中进行数据复验。基于临床试验电子数据管理系统（EDC）进行数据管理的，还需要提交注释病例报告表。

原始数据库和分析数据库可以 Excel 形式进行递交，但应注意，行政相对人不应仅递交一个与临床申报资料中的数据汇总表一致的 Excel 表格，还应按照上述要求递交分析数据库、说明性文件。

第四章

其他技术共性问题

107. 问：采用同品种或临床试验路径进行临床评价的产品，审评过程中被列入《免于临床评价医疗器械目录》，申请人补充资料时是否可免于进行临床评价？

答： 在审医疗器械采用同品种临床评价或临床试验路径进行临床评价的，如在申请人提交注册申报资料后，申报产品列入正式发布的《免于临床评价医疗器械目录》，申请人在补充资料时可根据其需要，按照《列入免于进行临床评价医疗器械目录产品对比说明技术指导原则》，从基本原理、结构组成、性能、安全性、适用范围等方面，证明产品的安全有效性。此种情形下，考虑到补充资料中的临床评价资料与首次递交时相比，发生较大变化，申请人可充分利用发补后咨询和预审查等沟通交流路径，与审评人员进行充分沟通。

108. 问：体外辅助生殖用液类产品是否可选择同品种临床评价路径开展临床评价？

答： 部分体外辅助生殖用液类产品已列入《免于临床评价医疗器械目录》。不在该目录的体外辅助生殖用液类产品，建议结合申报产品实际特点及可提供的支持资料情况，选择合适的临床评价路径，包括临床试验和同品种临床评价路径。如企业拟通过同品种临床评价路径申报注册，可考虑如下情况后进行综合评价。

（1）考虑到体外辅助生殖用液类产品组分多样，在针对组分进行对比时，如选定的单一同品种产品组分不能覆盖申报产品的所有组分，可以考虑增加同品种器械，以支持单一同品种未能覆盖的申报产品组分。

（2）对于生理盐成分、能量底物、酸碱缓冲体系、氨基酸、人血清白蛋白、抗生素等常见基础组分浓度的差异，如无法获得同品种各组分浓度，且以上成分浓度差异对安全、有效性的影响可通过性能指标的对比体现，如 pH、渗透压、杂质限量、使用性能指标、鼠胚试验等指标的对比，可不提供浓度对比信息。与预期用途相关的特殊功能性组分需提供浓度对比信息，并评价差异性对安全有效性的影响。

（3）进行同品种临床评价时，使用临床文献数据、临床经验数据时应注意评价指标应能反映产品的临床用途，体现产品相关的临床结局，如包含受精率、卵裂率、囊胚率、着床率、妊娠率等适用的指标。

109. 问：采用光学跟踪和（或）电磁跟踪技术，用于引导经皮置针或跟踪导航手术器械的手术导航系统是否必须提供基于临床试验的临床评价资料？

答： 此类产品是否需要开展临床试验可结合产品的临床功能、适用范围、现有非临床验证的充分性以及境内已获准上市产品的情况等方面综合判定。例如以下两类产品可考虑采用同品种对比路径开展临床评价。

（1）包含持针机械臂的患者术前影像引导胸腹部的经皮置针（包括活检针、消融针）。机械臂可按照医生确认的置针路径完成置针的功能。

（2）不包含机械臂的跟踪导航手术器械。具有术前对手术器械的入路规划、多模态影像配准/融合等功能，可根据患者术前影像引导医师实施外科手术操作。

采用同品种对比路径开展临床评价时，建议充分对比与分析，申报产品与同品种产品在临床功能、性能参数等方面异同的基础上，考虑提供台架试验、动物试验、同类产品临床文献等资料论证产品的安全有效性，必要时也可考虑提供符合相关管理要求的尸体研究数据。

110. 问：行政相对人采用境外临床试验数据开展临床评价时，申请人是否仍需在中国境内开展临床试验？

答:《接受医疗器械境外临床试验数据技术指导原则》第五条中已明确"若特定医疗器械的技术审评指导原则中含有对其临床试验的相关要求，该器械境外临床试验应考虑有关要求，存在不一致时，应提供充分、合理的理由和依据"。因此，若申请人已经按照《接受医疗器械境外临床试验数据技术指导原则》提交了符合伦理、依法、科学原则的临床试验数据，且充分考虑了技术审评要求的差异、受试人群的差异、临床试验条件差异，可不在中国境内额外开展临床试验。

111. 问：申请髋关节假体产品注册，如何选择临床评价路径？如选择同品种临床评价路径，需关注哪些内容？

答: 申请髋关节假体产品注册，可结合申报产品具体的适用范围和技术特征，选择合适的临床评价路径。一般来说，如已有相同适用范围、相似技术特征（如作用机理、材料、设计、产品性能等）的同品种产品在国内上市，行政相对人可考虑通过同品种路径进行临床评价。

髋关节假体进行同品种临床评价时，需符合《医疗器械临床评价技术指导原则》的适用部分，建议关注如下事项。

（1）同品种产品的选择尽量选择适用范围相同、技术特征与申报产品相同或尽可能相似的境内已上市产品作为同品种产品。如果选择的同品种产品与申报产品差异较大，则需提供更多的科学证据论证二者差异不对产品安全有效性产生不利影响。鼓励申请人选择同品种产品时，对已上市同类产品进行全面调研。

（2）申报产品与同品种产品的对比需明确申报产品和同品种产品的范围相同和技术特征，详述二者的相同性和差异性。

（3）同品种产品临床数据的提供申请人需明确临床数据与同品种产品的相关性。建议申请人提取临床文献中的关键要素，以便于后续数据分析。

（4）差异部分科学证据的提供根据申报产品与同品种产品的具体差异，需提交恰当的科学证据，如申报产品的非临床研究资料和（或）临床数据，包括可代表申报产品的非临床研究资料和（或）临床数据。

112. 问：行政相对人在试验过程中多次修订临床试验方案，提交产品注册时，是否需提交历次试验方案、伦理委员会意见、知情同意书？

答： 如涉及临床试验方案的修订，行政相对人需提交最终版本的临床试验方案、知情同意书和历次临床试验方案变更的伦理委员会意见和变更理由。

最终版本的临床试验方案，应详细列明历次变更情况；如未列明，则需提交历次变更的临床试验方案。

113. 问：申报产品的所有型号规格是否均需进行临床试验？

答： 应结合申报产品型号规格的差异，综合评估临床试验使用型号规格是否可代表申报产品的所有型号规格，建议基于申报产品适用范围、临床试验目的、评价指标等，分析申报产品各型号间差异。如临床试验使用型号规格可代表申报产品的所有型号规格，则不需要使用所有型号规格进行临床试验。

114. 问：如某产品的临床试验方案中包括可行性试验和确证性试验，试验结束后，是否可将可行性试验和确证性临床试验的结果合并统计？

答： 可行性试验可初步评估产品的安全性和性能，为确证性试验设计提供信息，其与确证性临床试验的目的不同。试验结果的统计，应遵循预先规定的统计分析计划。不建议在试验结束后，将可行性试验和确证性临床试验结果合并统计。

115. 问：已注册产品如未能在规定时间内申请延续注册，按照法规要求，需申请产品注册。此时，临床评价可否选择原注册产品作为同品种产品，完成临床评价？临床数据应该如何提供？

答：此种情形下，可选择原注册产品作为同品种产品，完成临床评价。同品种对比主要关注申报产品与原注册产品是否存在差异，如二者不存在差异，可提供该产品上市前和上市后的临床数据，以及上市后不良事件在内的临床经验数据。

116. 问：医疗器械（不含体外诊断试剂产品）产品指导原则中若要求某产品在具有境外临床试验数据的基础上仍需在中国境内开展临床试验，而申请人已经按照《接受医疗器械境外临床试验数据技术指导原则》提交了符合三条基本原则的临床试验数据，并且充分考虑了技术审评要求的差异、受试人群的差异、临床试验条件差异，是否可不在中国境内开展临床试验？

答：可以。《接受医疗器械境外临床试验技术指导原则》第五条中已明确"若特定医疗器械的技术审评指导原则中含有对其临床试验的相关要求，该器械境外临床试验应考虑有关要求，存在不一致时，应提供充分、合理的理由和依据"。因此，若能够说明境外临床试验数据结论可外推至中国使用人群，且符合中国注册相关技术要求，其数据即可用于临床评价，不需再在中国境内开展临床试验。

117. 问：单组目标值医疗器械临床试验设计中，目标值的定义和构建原则是什么？

答：与目标值比较的单组设计需事先指定主要评价指标有临床意义的目标值，通过考察单组临床试验主要评价指标的结果是否在指定的目标值范围内，从而评价试验器械有效性 / 安全性。由于没有设置对照组，单组目标值设计的临床试验无法确证试验器械的优效、等效或非劣效，仅能确证试验器械的有效性 / 安全性达到专业领域内公认的最低标准。

目标值是专业领域内公认的某类医疗器械的有效性 / 安全性评价指标所应达到的最低标准，包括客观性能标准（objective performance criteria，OPC）和性能目标（performance goal，PG）两种。目标值通常为二分类（如有效 / 无效）指标，也可为定量指标，包括靶值和单侧置信区间界限（通常为 97.5% 单侧置信区间界限）。对临床试验结果进行统计分析时，需计算主要评价指标的点估计值和单侧置信区间界限值，并将其与目标值进行比较。

目标值的构建通常需要全面收集具有一定质量水平及相当数量病例的临床研究数据，并进行科学分析（如 Meta 分析）。随着器械技术和临床技能的提高，OPC 可能发生改变，需要对临床数据重新进行分析以确认。

118. 问：应如何考虑基于深度学习的计算机辅助决策产品临床试验设计类型？

答： 基于深度学习的计算机辅助决策产品一般分为两类。

（1）对患者是否患有目标疾病，从而对患者的分诊转诊提供辅助决策建议的产品。该类产品不给出具体病变情况，且无论辅助分诊结果为阴性、阳性，均需专业医师再一次对患者影像进行评阅，如糖尿病视网膜病变辅助分诊、肺炎辅助分诊、脑出血辅助分诊等各类目标疾病患者的计算机辅助分诊、转诊产品等。该类产品的临床试验设计可以考虑采用单组目标值设计，主要评价指标为产品辅助分诊结果的诊断准确度指标（如敏感度、特异度等，通常为患者水平）。

（2）对目标疾病的病变病灶进行辅助检测的产品，如肺结节辅助检测产品、骨折 CT 影像辅助检测产品等。该类产品的临床试验建议采用对照设计，试验组为医师与申报产品共同检测，对照组为传统检测诊断方法（如临床医师的阅片/综合诊断）。主要评价指标为诊断准确度指标（如敏感度、特异度、AFROC 曲线、检出率等，一般灵敏度考虑病灶病变水平，特异度考虑患者水平）。临床试验比较类型应能够体现产品受益风险的可接受性，建议考虑优效性设计，如针对 4mm 以上肺结节 CT 影像辅助检测软件可考虑患者水平的特异度为优效和病灶水平的敏感度为非劣效。

119. 问：最高可闭合 7mm 血管的超声软组织切割止血系统的注册申报资料是否可以体外爆破压试验和动物试验资料代替临床评价资料？

答：根据《超声软组织切割止血系统同品种临床评价技术审查指导原则》，由于最高可闭合 7mm 血管的超声软组织切割止血系统临床使用风险相对较高、技术难度相对较大，建议在体外爆破压试验和动物试验的基础之上，通过申报产品自身临床数据进一步论证其安全有效性。在境内开展的临床试验应符合《医疗器械临床试验质量管理规范》相关要求。

120. 问：颅内药物涂层球囊扩张导管临床试验时是否可以选择单组目标值设计？

答：单组目标值设计的实质是将主要评价指标的试验结果与已有临床数据进行比较，以评价试验器械的有效性 / 安全性。与平行对照试验相比，单组试验的固有偏倚是非同期对照偏倚，由于时间上的不同步，可能引起选择偏倚、混杂偏倚、测量偏倚和评价偏倚等。由于没有设置对照组，单组目标值设计的临床试验无法确证试验器械的优效、等效或非劣效，仅能确证试验器械的有效性 / 安全性达到专业领域内公认的最低标准。当试验器械技术比较成熟且对其适用疾病有较为深刻的了解时，或者当设置对照在客观上不可行时（例如试验器械与现有治疗方法的风险受益过于悬殊，设置对照在伦理上不可行；又如现有治疗方法因客观条件限制不具有可行性等），方可考虑采用单组目标值设计。

根据颅内药物涂层球囊扩张导管的技术发展和临床应用现状，不符合单组目标值设计的基本原则，建议选择 RCT 试验设计进行临床试验。

121. 问：全缝线锚钉如何通过同品种对比开展临床评价？

答：全缝线锚钉可通过同品种对比开展临床评价，同品种器械应选择具有相同适用范围的已获准境内上市同类产品。

与同品种医疗器械的对比项目包括设计原理、结构组成、尺寸规格、操作性能、力学性能等。结构尺寸对比需包括自然状态下和软锚收缩后结构尺寸对比，明确编织方式以及单股线的粗细等异同。针对结构尺寸差异，需解释申报产品选择该设计的原因，并结合后续力学性能证明差异不对产品安全有效性产生不利影响。操作性能对比包括插入力、软锚收缩是否容易成结等，对于非定量的操作性能评价指标，产品设计验证资料显示可满足临床需求时，可不需与同品种产品进行对比。力学性能对比包括动静态固定性能的对比，申报产品的力学性能不应差于同品种产品。在与同品种器械进行力学性能对比时，需注意试验参数（如荷载大小和循环次数等）和力学测试固定块选择的合理性。若使用人工骨，建议根据临床使用情形下的骨质条件确定模拟块构成（如皮质骨/松质骨复合块）、厚度和密度等，测试钻孔直径大小与临床使用时的直径保持一致。在提供各力学测试报告时，需注意明确各试样失效模式。

对于预期应用在生物力学要求显著不同的解剖部位的锚钉，需分别与具有相同适用范围的锚钉进行对比。

122. 问：临床试验是否需针对同一注册单元所有型号规格进行试验？

答：原则上应考虑产品工作原理、适用范围、型号规格间区别及非临床研究数据，并结合临床试验的研究目的、主要评价指标等，综合考量后确认进行临床试验的产品是否具有典型性，能覆盖申报产品的所有型号规格。

123. 问：经导管心脏瓣膜及输送系统已进行临床试验并在境内上市，之后在经导管心脏瓣膜未发生变化的情况下，仅针对其输送系统进行了改进，应适合选择哪种临床路径进行申报？

答：行政相对人应具体分析输送系统的变化对产品性能及临床安全性是否存在影响，同时重点分析临床前研究数据是否足以支持差异不对产品安全有效性产生影响。如分析评价后风险可接受，且非临床资料及境外同类产品具有相同改进应用的临床数据可以支持输送系统的变更，行政相对人可选择同品种路径进行临床评价。

124. 问：拟通过临床试验进行临床评价时，是否需要以及如何提交临床评价报告？

答： 需要提交临床评价报告，可以根据《医疗器械注册申报临床评价报告技术指导原则》"四、通过临床试验获取的临床数据进行临床评价"要求进行临床评价，并参考"五、临床评价报告的参考格式"要求提供临床评价报告。

125. 问：递交境外临床试验资料进行临床评价时，是否需要递交临床试验原始数据资料？

答： 递交境外临床试验资料进行临床评价需符合《接受医疗器械境外临床试验数据技术指导原则》相关要求，并按照《医疗器械临床试验数据递交要求注册审查指导原则》递交临床试验数据资料，包括原始数据库、分析数据库、说明性文件和代码等。

126. 问：已有境外医疗器械临床试验数据的产品，如境内也有已发布的相应产品的临床试验指导原则，此时产品境外临床试验数据是否必须完全满足境内相应指导原则要求？

答： 境外进行的临床试验可能符合试验开展所在国家（地区）的技术审评要求，但不一定完全符合我国相关审评要求。例如进行临床试验设计时，有些国家仅要求临床试验能够得出器械性能达到某一观察终点的结论；但在我国申报注册时，可能要求该器械性能达到多个观察终点才可确认其有效性，且医疗器械的安全性有适当的证据支持。若国家药品监督管理局发布特定医疗器械的技术审评指导原则中含有对其临床试验的相关要求，该器械境外临床试验应考虑有关要求，存在不一致时，应提供充分、合理的理由和依据。

127. 问：如何选择医疗器械临床评价路径？

答：《医疗器械监督管理条例》规定，开展医疗器械临床评价，可以根据产品特征、临床风险、已有临床数据等情形，通过开展临床试验，或者通过对同品种医疗器械临床文献资料、临床数据进行分析评价，证明医疗器械的安全性、有效性。注册申请人可参照《决策是否开展医疗器械临床试验技术指导原则》判定是否需要开展临床试验，并结合近期国家药监局医疗器械技术审评中心（以下简称器审中心）发布的"《医疗器械分类目录》子目录相关产品临床评价推荐路径"的通告，选择适宜的临床评价路径。

128. 问：按照同品种医疗器械临床数据进行临床评价时，如检索不到同品种医疗器械的临床文献怎么办？

答：同品种医疗器械临床数据的收集、分析与评价，根据申报产品设计特点、关键技术、适用范围和风险程度的不同，具有不同作用，包括确认同品种医疗器械的安全有效性是否已得到临床公认，风险受益是否在可接受范围内；充分识别同品种医疗器械的临床使用风险，为申报产品的风险受益分析提供信息；通过临床数据确认非临床研究的剩余风险；为部分非临床研究（如台架试验）测试结果的评价提供临床数据等。

同品种产品临床数据除了临床文献数据，还包括临床经验数据和临床试验数据，临床经验数据包括已完成的临床研究数据集、不良事件数据集和与临床风险相关的纠正措施数据集，其中不良事件数据集可以通过监管机构上市后的投诉、不良事件公开获取。

此外，申请人还需确认选取的同品种产品是否为同类产品中临床关注度较高的、安全有效性已得到公认的产品，以及文献检索策略是否恰当，能否保证检索的全面性。

129. 问：下腔静脉滤器临床试验主要评价指标需要考虑哪些因素？

答：下腔静脉滤器（IVCF）是为预防下腔静脉系统深静脉血栓形成（DVT）的栓子脱落引起肺动脉栓塞（PE）而设计的一种装置。下腔静脉滤器植入期间滤器的位置、形态不仅影响过滤栓子的效果，也与使用风险密切相关，比如植入期间滤器发生位移、倾斜、血管壁发生穿孔的情况，不仅降低栓子过滤效果，也可能增加不良事件风险。因此主要评价指标一般需要综合考虑上述因素，至少包含患者肺栓塞发生率和滤器的位置、形态等。

130. 问：个性化基台或可切削基台柱选择同品种比对路径进行临床评价时，应选择什么类型基台作为同品种产品。

答： 个性化基台或可切削基台柱与配用种植体的接口一般是固定接口，申请人可以选择配用种植体对应的成品基台作为同品种器械进行对比例如三角形、六边形、梅花形等接口类型中，每种类型至少分别选择一个成品基台进行同品种比对。一般不选择其他个性化基台或可切削基台柱作为同品种产品，但可作为可比器械，与申报产品对比可切削范围。

131. 问：颅内抽吸导管在开展同品种比对时，动物试验中对血管和血栓类型的选择需要注意哪些方面？

答： 动物试验建议从血管直径、血管迂曲度、血管壁特征等方面论述所选择血管的代表性。以猪模型为例，可以考虑选择咽升动脉、颈外动脉、颈总动脉，舌动脉，锁骨下动脉以及其他适宜的血管。申请人应逐一说明靶血管的选择理由和依据，所选择的血管应至少包括1个以上为受试动物颅内供血的血管，并考虑产品拟宣称使用的最小直径血管以及迂曲度较大的血管。人工血栓应考虑制作不同类型的血栓，常用类型包括软血栓、混合型血栓、硬血栓。其中混合型血栓可作为软血栓的代表模型。

132. 问：创新医疗器械特别审查申请表中备注栏有哪些填写要求？

答：行政相对人应完整填写创新医疗器械特别审查申请表备注内容，要求如下：行政相对人如实填写利益相关方面的专家/单位信息，包括并不限于理化指标检测、生物性能试验、动物试验、临床试验、合作研究者、知识产权买卖方等，并明确申请回避的专家及理由。如有涉及利益相关的专家，应明确专家参与的具体企业的名称及具体研发项目名称。备注信息不能为空，如无相关内容可填写"无"。

133. 问：创新医疗器械特别审查对提交的知识产权证明文件有哪些要求？

答：根据《创新医疗器械特别审查程序》中的有关规定，创新医疗器械特别审查中提交的知识产权证明文件应满足以下要求。

（1）行政相对人已获取中国发明专利权的，需提供经行政相对人签章的专利授权证书、权利要求书、说明书复印件和专利主管部门出具的专利登记簿副本原件。创新医疗器械特别审查申请时间距专利授权公告日不超过 5 年。

（2）行政相对人依法通过受让取得在中国发明专利使用权的，除提交专利权人持有的专利授权证书、权利要求书、说明书、专利登记簿副本复印件外，还需提供经专利主管部门出具的《专利实施许可合同备案证明》原件。创新医疗器械特别审查申请时间距专利授权公告日不超过 5 年。

（3）发明专利申请已由国务院专利行政部门公开、未获得授权的，需提供经行政相对人签章的发明专利已公开证明文件（如发明专利申请公布通知书、发明专利申请公布及进入实质审查阶段通知书、发明专利申请进入实质审查阶段通知书等）复印件和公布版本的权利要求书、说明书复印件。由国家知识产权局专利检索咨询中心出具检索报告，报告载明产品核心技术方案具备新颖性和创造性。发明专利申请审查过程中，权利要求书和说明书应专利审查部门要求发生修改的，需提交修改文本；专利权人发生变更的，提交专利主管部门出具的证明性文件，如手续合格通知书复印件。

134. 问：进口产品申报创新医疗器械特别审查申请时对签章有什么要求？

答：进口创新医疗器械特别审查申请申报资料若无特别说明，原文资料均应由行政相对人签章，中文资料由代理人签章。原文资料"签章"是指：行政相对人的法定代表人或者负责人签名，或者签名并加盖组织机构印章，并且应当提交由行政相对人所在地公证机构出具的公证件；中文资料"签章"是指：代理人盖公章，或者其法定代表人、负责人签名并加盖公章。关于资料公证的要求请参考《国家药监局关于医疗器械电子申报有关资料要求的通告》中的有关规定。

135. 问：创新医疗器械特别审查的时限及如何查询创新申报结果？

答： 根据《创新医疗器械特别审查程序》中的有关规定，创新医疗器械审查办公室收到创新医疗器械特别审查申请后，应当于 60 个工作日内出具审查意见（公示及异议处理时间不计算在内）。对拟进行特别审查的申请项目，应当在国家药监局医疗器械技术审评中心网站将行政相对人、产品名称予以公示，公示时间应当不少于 10 个工作日。对于公示内容有异议的，应当对相关意见研究后作出最终审查决定。行政相对人可通过登录国家药监局医疗器械技术审评中心网站审评进度查询页面来查询审查结果。

136. 问：境内创新医疗器械特别审查申请受理审核时对省局初审证明文件的要求是什么？

答： 境内行政相对人应当向其所在地的省级药品监督管理部门提出创新医疗器械特别审查申请（以下称创新申请）。省级药品监督管理部门对申报项目是否符合《创新医疗器械特别审查程序》第二条要求进行初审。行政相对人在创新申请时，应提交经省局初审的相关证明文件。若创新申请在受理审核过程中受理补正，行政相对人对受理补正问题完成补充后再次提交时，可不再进行省局初审，同时提交前次省局初审的相关证明文件作为省局初审凭证。对于受理后已经出具审查意见，再次申请创新医疗器械特别审查的项目，需再次经省局初审，并提交经省局初审的相关证明文件。

137. 问：境内第三类医疗器械／体外诊断试剂质量管理体系核查工作时限有什么规定？

答： 根据《医疗器械注册与备案管理办法》及《体外诊断试剂注册与备案管理办法》中的有关规定，境内第三类医疗器械／体外诊断试剂质量管理体系核查时限如下。

（1）器审中心应当在医疗器械／体外诊断试剂注册申请资料起 10 个工作日内，通知相应省、自治区、直辖市药品监督管理部门开展注册质量管理体系核查。

（2）省、自治区、直辖市药品监督管理部门原则上应当自收到体系核查通知后 30 个工作日内完成核查，并将核查情况、核查结果等相关材料反馈至器审中心。

138. 问：按照《医疗器械注册人制度》生产的境内第三类产品注册质量管理体系，体系核查通知的发送及体系核查结果文件的出具有什么要求？

答： 根据《关于进一步做好第三类医疗器械注册人试点工作的通知》中的相关要求，体系核查通知仅发至行政相对人（委托人）所在地药品监督管理部门；体系核查结果文件由行政相对人（委托人）所在地药品监督管理部门，发送至国家药监局技术审评机构，所出具的体系核查结果报告中应当注明受托企业名称、生产地址等信息。

139. 问：专家咨询会如果需要行政相对人参会，行政相对人的参会的形式是什么？

答： 根据《医疗器械技术审评中心专家咨询会 / 专家公开论证会操作规范》中的相关要求，参加专家咨询会的人员仅限于与会专家和相关审评人员。如需行政相对人参会的，行政相对人以在线方式候会，主审人汇总会上提出的问题，通过一个端口以视频会议方式连线行政相对人，进行现场解答，问题解答完行政相对人即退场。

140. 问：专家咨询会会议时限及行政相对人回避时间的要求是什么？

答： 根据《医疗器械技术审评中心专家咨询会 / 专家公开论证会操作规范》的相关要求，在行政相对人收到《关于召开专家咨询会相关事项的通知》后，境内产品于 30 个工作日内召开会议，进口产品于 40 个工作日内召开会议。

若有特殊情况，行政相对人可提供会议回避日期，回避日期应当在接到本通知的规定时间内（境内产品 30 个工作日，进口产品 40 个工作日）。回避时间超出规定时间范围之外的，行政相对人应提出延期申请并说明理由，申请延期时间不超过 20 个工作日。

141. 问：专家咨询会的会议议程是什么？

答： 根据《医疗器械技术审评中心专家咨询会／专家公开论证会操作规范》的相关要求，主持人宣布会议开始，会议原则上按以下议程进行：

（1）综合业务部人员播放行政相对人录制的 PPT 视频；

（2）主审人与专家进行相关问题讨论，并由主审人汇总问题；

（3）行政相对人线上进入会场，主审宣读汇总问题，行政相对人进行答辩，答辩结束后行政相对人离场；

（4）专家评议并提出咨询会审意见（申请人回避），认真填写《专家咨询会咨询意见表》；

（5）主审人确认咨询问题已获得明确意见，并协助组长整理会审意见。

142. 问：国家药监局医疗器械技术审评中心在医疗器械注册审评工作中，可召开专家咨询会的条件有哪些？

答： 根据《医疗器械技术审评中心专家咨询会／专家公开论证会操作规范》的要求，属下列情形之一的，经各分技术委员会讨论通过后可召开专家咨询会：

（1）通过创新审查的医疗器械；

（2）通过优先审批的医疗器械；

（3）通过应急审批的医疗器械；

（4）同品种首个的医疗器械；

（5）临床试验审批申请。

其他产品在审评中的技术问题，由各分技术委员会自行研究解决，存在争议的可提交中心技术委员会讨论，确需咨询专家意见的经中心技术委员会同意后可由审评员提出专家咨询会申请。

143. 问：专家咨询会会前告知行政相对人的程序是什么？

答：根据《医疗器械技术审评中心专家咨询会 / 专家公开论证会操作规范》的相关要求，专家咨询会会前告知行政相对人的程序如下。

（1）对于需要行政相对人参会的，综合业务部收到专家咨询会申请批件后，应当在 2 个工作日内，向行政相对人发送《关于召开专家咨询会相关事项的通知》，并负责收取回执。行政相对人在收到通知后，应当在 5 个工作日内将回执反馈至综合业务部，并在回执中明确回避会议时间、理由，以及行政相对人外请参会专家名单，如需回避有利益冲突的专家，应当说明回避理由并提供真实证据。

（2）综合业务部在向行政相对人发出《关于召开专家咨询会相关事项的通知》后，5 个工作日内未收到回执或因行政相对人提供的信息错误而导致综合业务部无法发送《关于召开专家咨询会相关事项的通知》的，综合业务部直接按时限要求安排专家咨询会。

（3）对于不需要行政相对人参会的，综合业务部直接按时限要求安排专家咨询会。

144. 问：国家标准品发生更新，何种情形下已注册体外诊断试剂无需办理变更注册？

答： 根据中国食品药品检定研究院（以下简称"中检院"）对体外诊断试剂国家标准品的管理，国家标准品的批号是由"品种编号（6位数字）＋批号（6位数字）"组成，在中检院官方网站对外公布，可查询。国家标准品的更新包括"换批"与"换代"两种情况，其区别在于："换批"是为了保证国家标准品供应量而制备的新批次，国家标准品的设置、量值和性能接受标准均未发生变化，品种编号不变，仅批号发生变化；"换代"则表明国家标准品整体发生变化，其设置、量值或者性能接受标准均可能发生改变，品种编号和批号均发生变化。据此，国家标准品发生更新而无需办理变更注册的情形包括：

（1）医疗器械（体外诊断试剂）注册证有效期内有国家标准品发生"换批"更新时，无需办理变更注册，但应当在延续注册申报资料中对延续注册产品符合国家标准品的相关情况给予说明。

（2）医疗器械（体外诊断试剂）注册证有效期内有国家标准品发生"换代"更新，已注册产品的注册证及其附件载明事项均不发生变化，或者仅更新引用的国家标准品品种编号及批号，即符合新的国家标准品要求，则无需办理变更注册。具体包括以下两种情形。

1）申报产品有适用的国家标准品：产品技术要求或说明书直接引用"国家标准品的说明书条款内容"或者"国家标准品品

种编号＋批号"。国家标准品"换代"更新，品种编号及批号发生变化，涉及引用的国家标准品的说明书条款内容未发生变化。

2）申报产品无适用的国家标准品：产品技术要求或说明书参考引用某个"国家标准品的说明书条款内容"或者"国家标准品品种编号＋批号"。国家标准品"换代"更新，品种编号及批号发生变化，涉及参考引用的国家标准品的说明书条款内容未发生变化；或者涉及参考引用的国家标准品的说明书条款内容发生变化，但产品技术要求或说明书仍参考引用更新前的国家标准品相关内容。

145. 问：行政相对人完全不具备自检能力或只有部分自检能力，如完全或者部分委托有资质的检测机构进行检测，是否可以同时委托多个有资质的检测机构进行检测？

答： 行政相对人若不具备产品技术要求中全部条款或部分条款项目的检验能力，可以将相关条款项目委托一家或多家有资质的医疗器械检验机构进行检验，注册申请人应当确保委托检验样品的一致性。（对于产品技术要求完全采用国家标准、行业标准的，检验机构必须取得该国家标准、行业标准的资质认定，报告封面加盖资质认定标志 CMA 章，并在报告备注中注明；对于产品技术要求不涉及或部分涉及国家标准、行业标准进行检验并出具报告的，应在检验报告书备注中对承检能力予以自我表明，并承担相应的法律责任。）提交注册申请时，注册申请人应当根据委托检验结果形成自检报告，所有的委托检验报告应作为自检报告附件一并提交。

146. 问：进口医疗器械已在中国境内获得注册证，现拟由境外转移至境内生产，应如何申请注册？

答：依据《国家药品监督管理局关于实施〈医疗器械注册与备案管理办法〉〈体外诊断试剂注册与备案管理办法〉有关事项的通告》，境外企业在境内生产的医疗器械，应当由境内生产的企业作为注册申请人（备案人）申请注册（办理备案）。已获得注册证的进口器械，可以参考《国家药监局关于进口医疗器械产品在中国境内企业生产有关事项的公告》提交注册申报资料。

147. 问：对于境内刚成立的医疗器械生产企业，在研发过程中遇到技术问题时，是否可以申请注册受理前技术问题咨询？

答：依据《关于医疗器械审评检查长三角、大湾区分中心开展审评业务及器审中心咨询工作安排调整的通告》，咨询对象应为境内医疗器械研制机构、生产企业，法人证书或营业执照范围中包含医疗器械生产，可以申请注册受理前技术问题咨询。

148. 问：境外行政相对人在华常驻代表处、办事处能作为境外申请人、备案人的代理人吗？

答：依据《医疗器械注册与备案管理办法》第十四条、《体外诊断试剂注册与备案管理办法》第十五条要求，境外申请人、备案人应当指定中国境内的企业法人作为代理人，办理相关医疗器械 / 体外诊断试剂注册、备案事项。代理人应当依法协助注册人、备案人履行《医疗器械监督管理条例》第二十条第一款规定的义务，并协助境外注册人、备案人落实相应法律责任。

按照上述要求，境外行政相对人在华常驻代表处、办事处不能作为代理人。

149. 问：如行政相对人没有 CA 证书，该如何提交国产第三类、进口第二类、第三类医疗器械注册及创新医疗器械特别审查相关文件？受理补正后的文件该如何递交？

答： 请按照《关于公布医疗器械注册申报资料要求和批准证明文件格式的公告》《关于公布体外诊断试剂注册申报资料要求和批准证明文件格式的公告》《国家药监局关于发布创新医疗器械特别审查程序的公告》的法规要求将纸质资料、电子版资料（U 盘内容：上传资料文件夹、文件夹压缩包及一致性声明）及具体办理人提交的行政相对人或其代理人授权书及其身份证复印件准备完善，并寄送至国家药监局受理大厅。国家药监局医疗器械技术审评中心工作人员将为行政相对人办理资料上传。经受理审查，需要行政相对人补正的，国家药监局医疗器械技术审评中心将通过 EMS 将受理补正通知和纸质资料一并寄回，行政相对人根据受理补正意见完善后需要再次申请的，应当按照线下方式办理。

行政相对人获得 CA 证书后，可通过 eRPS 系统自行提交注册申请、办理补正资料预审查、提交补正资料等业务，但在取得 CA 证书前已通过线下途径提交且已受理的注册申请，仍应通过线下途径办理完毕，不可通过 CA 证书线上途径办理。

150. 问：如何有效地与受理大厅沟通受理通知书 / 补正通知书 / 备案凭证等相关纸质资料准确的快递地址及联系人信息？

答：受理大厅会优先以申请表其他需要说明的问题中备注的快递地址及联系人信息作为有效快递信息，如此部分无内容，则以申请表中申请人 / 注册人 / 代理人信息作为有效快递信息。为确保相关文书及时准确送达，建议准确填写注册申请表。

151. 问：如何判断申请延续注册时间是否在医疗器械注册证有效期届满 6 个月前？

答：医疗器械注册证有效期届满需要延续注册的，注册人应当在医疗器械注册证有效期届满 6 个月前申请延续注册，并按照相关要求提交申请资料。因申请资料不齐全或者不符合法定形式需要补正资料，器审中心将在受理补正通知中注明注册人首次申请延续注册时间。注册人补正后再次申请延续注册时，应当提交受理补正通知，器审中心将根据受理补正通知中注明的注册人首次申请延续注册时间判定申请延续注册时间是否在医疗器械注册证有效期届满 6 个月前，并按照《医疗器械注册与备案管理办法》规定对申请资料进行审核。

152. 问：已注册医疗器械（体外诊断试剂）产品技术要求引用的强制性标准内容发生变化，何种情形下无需办理变更注册？

答： 医疗器械注册证有效期内有新的强标发布实施，已注册产品的注册证及其附件载明事项均不发生变化，即符合新的强标，具体包括以下两种情形。

（1）产品技术要求引用强标的形式为"直接引用强制性标准条款具体内容"、"标准编号"或者"标准编号＋年代号"。强标更新，标准编号和／或年代号发生变化，但产品技术要求引用的强标条款内容未发生变化。

（2）产品技术要求直接参考引用了某个强标的条款内容，强标更新，但产品技术要求参考引用的强标条款内容未发生变化；或者产品技术要求参考引用的强标条款内容发生变化，但产品技术要求仍参考引用更新前的强标条款内容。

上述两种情形下，产品技术要求不发生变化或者仅更新引用的标准编号和（或）年代号，无需单独办理变更注册。

153. 问：《中国药典》是否属于医疗器械强制性标准？产品技术要求中关于"无菌"的性能指标、检验方法，已经符合 2015 版《中国药典》，是否需要升级符合 2020 版《中国药典》？

答： 中国药典不属于医疗器械强制性标准。如产品有适用的强制性标准，该强制性标准引用《中国药典》且未注明版本号，如注册人需要将产品技术要求中关于《中国药典》的内容更新至 2020 版，需要办理变更注册，获得变更文件后再申请延续注册；如产品有适用的强制性标准，该强制性标准引用《中国药典》且明确版本号为 2015 版，或无菌检验引用的《中国药典》未涉及被强制性标准引用，或产品无强制性标准，可按无菌检验符合 2015 版中国药典无变化延续。

154. 问：已注册医疗器械（体外诊断试剂）产品本身没有任何变化，仅产品适用的强制性标准更新，能否提交符合新的强制性标准的检测报告，申报延续注册？

答： 延续注册引用的强制性标准若涉及其具体条款变化，建议单独提交变更注册申请取得原审批部门批准的变更注册文件后，再提出延续注册申请。但注册人应当在医疗器械注册证有效期届满 6 个月前申请延续注册，并按照相关要求提交申请资料。因申请资料不齐全或者不符合法定形式需要补正资料，器审中心将在受理补正通知中注明注册人首次申请延续注册时间。注册人补正后再次申请延续注册时，应当提交受理补正通知，器审中心将根据受理补正通知中注明的注册人首次申请延续注册时间判定申请延续注册时间是否在医疗器械注册证有效期届满 6 个月前，并按照《医疗器械注册与备案管理办法》或《体外诊断试剂注册与备案管理办法》规定对申请资料进行审核。

155. 问：医疗器械主文档所有者或其代理机构进行主文档登记需使用 CA 证书，如何准备 CA 申领资料？

答： 自 2021 年 3 月 15 日起，境内主文档所有者或者进口主文档所有者委托的中国境内代理机构申领 CA（Certificate Authority）时需同时准备拟在主文档登记平台提交的《医疗器械主文档登记申请表》，经申领人盖章后与营业执照一同上传至"CA 证书申领"模块"1.5 企业营业执照副本扫描件"处。

156. 问：系统提示 CA 证书即将过期，该如何处理？

答： 首次申领 CA 证书后有效期为一年，当 CA 证书有效期不足 60 日时，系统将提示证书即将到期，如行政相对人希望继续使用 CA 证书，应于临近有效期前将 CA 插入电脑，登录"医疗器械注册企业服务平台"（https://erps.cmde.org.cn），点击"证书延续更新"并按照网页提示信息自行操作将有效期延续一年，具体操作流程见器审中心网站《关于医疗器械注册电子申报信息系统数字认证证书更新有关事宜的通知》。

157. 问：行政相对人是否可以在医疗器械注册证书或者变更文件正式下达前，对其中载明内容进行确认，减少注册证书及附件载明信息存在的错误情形？

答： 可以。在正式出具注册证书或变更文件前，器审中心会请行政相对人对注册证书或者变更文件及其附件（产品技术要求、说明书、以附页形式载明的注册证书或者变更文件信息）的内容进行确认。

对于线上项目，器审中心通过 eRPS 系统，将含有相应项目注册证书或者变更文件信息的《医疗器械注册证信息确认单》（以下简称《确认单》）及注册证书或者变更文件附件推送给行政相对人，行政相对人凭 CA 登录 eRPS 系统接收《确认单》，查看相应项目需确认内容并逐项进行核实，所有信息均完成确认后，点击"完成确认"按钮回复确认结果。如附件内容有误，还请行政相对人将确认后将最终版本附件的 PDF 文件通过电子邮件发送至审评员邮箱。线下项目通过电子邮件的形式发放《确认单》。详细操作见器审中心通告《关于开展医疗器械注册证书及其附件信息确认工作的通告》。

158. 问：若行政相对人发现已领取的注册证书、变更文件及其附件中存在需修正的内容，且该内容不属于实质性变更，原注册申报资料能够充分支持该修正的真实性、准确性和合理性，这种情况下行政相对人应该首选哪种修正方式？

答：行政相对人可以前往国家药品监督管理局行政事项受理服务和投诉举报中心制证处，向制证处工作人员说明情况并提出注册证信息修正申请，同时申领一份《注册证信息确认申请表》，将表中"申请人填写"部分填写完整，签字或盖章后交还给制证处工作人员。器审中心相应主审人收到《注册证信息确认申请表》后，第一时间对修正内容进行判断并将结果移交回制证处，行政相对人等待制证处通知，届时领取修正后的注册证书或变更文件及附件。

159. 问：医疗器械注册申请审评期间，对于拟作出不通过的审评结论的，器审中心是否会告知行政相对人，并提供提出异议的机会？

答： 在正式出具不予通过的审评结论前，器审中心会通过推送《医疗器械注册技术审评不通过结论确认单》（以下简称《确认单》），向行政相对人告知不通过的结论和理由，若行政相对人存在异议，应当自接到确认单之日起的 15 个工作日内提出，15 个工作日内未提出异议视为同意不通过的结论和理由。对于线上申报项目，通过 eRPS 系统完成《确认单》的推送及确认；线下项目通过电子邮件的形式发送《确认单》，对不通过的结论和理由有异议的，行政相对人邮件回复确认的同时，还需将经签章的纸质版《确认单》邮寄至器审中心相关人员。

器审中心收到异议后，对异议进行综合评估，并将异议评估结果以《医疗器械注册技术审评不通过结论异议综合评估意见告知单》的形式反馈至行政相对人，行政相对人无需对异议评估结果进行再次确认。

160. 问：立卷审查制度的定位是怎样的，与技术审评之间存在哪些差别？

答： 立卷审查指按照立卷审查要求对申报资料进行审查，对申报资料进入技术审评环节的完整性、合规性、一致性进行判断的过程。立卷审查不对产品的安全性、有效性、证明的合理性、充分性进行分析，亦不对产品风险受益比进行判定。立卷审查要求的实施使受理工作更加标准化、规范化，有利于提高进入审评环节的申报资料质量，降低审评发补率。

对于立卷审查要求中的问题，若在立卷审查环节未能做出充分判断，导致不应通过立卷审查环节的申报资料通过了立卷审查，在技术审评环节，仍可对立卷审查要求中的问题提出补正意见。

161. 问：在什么情形下，进口医疗器械产品在中国境内企业生产，可按照《国家药监局关于进口医疗器械产品在中国境内企业生产有关事项的公告》有关要求，准备注册申报资料？

答：当符合以下情形时，可以按照《国家药监局关于进口医疗器械产品在中国境内企业生产有关事项的公告》，部分注册申报资料可提交进口医疗器械的原注册申报资料。具体包括：

（1）进口医疗器械注册人通过其在境内设立的外商投资企业在境内生产第二类、第三类已获进口医疗器械注册证产品。

（2）中国境内企业投资的境外注册人在境内生产已获进口医疗器械注册证的第二类、第三类医疗器械产品的，由投资境外注册人的中国境内企业作为注册申请人申请该产品注册。

（3）我国香港、澳门、台湾地区已获医疗器械注册证的产品有关事项参照执行。

Chapter 1

Common technical issues of active medical device

1. Q: Can electrical stimulators and needle electrodes of equipment such as intraoperative electroencephalography (EEG) /electromyography (EMG) /evoked potential (EP) measurement system be applied for registration separately?

A: Electrical stimulators, needle electrodes and other accessories are generally required during the use of equipment such as intraoperative EEG/EMG/EP measurement system. Generally, electrical stimulator is integral to its connected equipment, and can be applied for registration together with the equipment. A needle electrode is generally provided in an independent aseptic package and intended for single use. As it is regulated as a medical device separately according to the *Classification Catalogue of Medical Devices*, it is recommended that it should be applied for registration separately.

2. Q: Does the X-ray image-guided system used in conjunction with the radiotherapy system need to be cooperatively tested with the radiotherapy system during a test?

A: Regarding the general-purpose image-guided system, a representative radiotherapy system should be selected for compatibility verification, relevant verification test data should be provided, and the reasons why the selected radiotherapy system is representative should be explained. In addition, relevant information such as general requirements, interface type of the radiotherapy system can be used in conjunction should also be clarified in the overview data.

A verification test should be performed for the dedicated image-guided system and the radiotherapy system used in conjunction. The relevant verification test data should be provided. In addition, relevant information such as manufacturer, model, Registration Certificate No. (a photocopy of the Registration Certificate should be provided) of the radiotherapy system used in conjunction should also be clarified in the overview data.

3. Q: If the medical X-ray diagnostic equipment is applicable to pediatric population, what study data should be submitted for this specific population?

A: Since children or newborns are very sensitive to X-ray, if the administrative counterpart declares that the equipment is suitable for pediatric population, it is necessary to provide the measures required to reduce the radiation dose for children or newborns. For example, automatic exposure control designed and calibrated for pediatric patients; protocol of low radiation dose suitable for children and infant; special filtration; incident radiation dosage lower than that for adults, prompt of exposure limit; displaying and recording the patient's dosage information or dose index as well as other patient information, such as age, height and weight (manual input or automatic calculation); grid which is demountable without use of tool.

4. Q: If reusable accessories are included in the registration unit when some active medical devices are applied for registration, what issues should be paid attention to in the disinfection and sterilization data of these accessories?

A: It should be ensured that the reusable accessories indeed have been disinfected or sterilized prior to use. The specific disinfection/sterilization methods (e.g. disinfectants and disinfection or sterilization equipment used) and important parameters of the disinfection/sterilization cycle (e.g. time, temperature and pressure) should be clarified in the Instructions for Use (IFU). The study data should include the following information: the determination basis of the disinfection/sterilization methods, the validation data of disinfection/sterilization effects and the research data related to the tolerance of the recommended disinfection/sterilization methods.

If there are many attachments of active medical devices, you can list the key information such as the name, model, use method, body contact, disinfection/sterilization method, and verification data number of the attachment to improve the readability of the data.

5. Q: As dentistry-powered polymerization activators generally contain light-guiding elements, what issues should be paid attention to during the test of the light-guiding elements?

A: If a powered polymerization activator has to be equipped with light-guiding elements during clinical use, it should be tested with the light-guiding elements, so as to evaluate whether it meets the requirements specified in 7.2 Radiation of YY 0055.1 or YY 0055.2. The types or models of the light-guiding elements selected for tests should cover all the light-guiding elements contained in the proposed product, or all the light-guiding elements that can be used in conjunction as specified in the accompanying documents. The types or models of the light-guiding elements should be reflected in the test report. The powered polymerization activator not intended to require light-guiding elements during use should be tested under normal use conditions.

6. Q: If changes only take place in power (including input power and/or the output power) during the change of registration of active equipment, is a full performance test required?

A: The full performance test is not required. The administrative counterpart should analyze which specific components of the proposed product are changed, describe the changes in detail in the overview data, and provide the verification data related to the changes in the study data. In addition to analyzing the impact of the changes on performance indicators, electrical safety and electromagnetic compatibility specified in the product technical specifications, the applicant should also be tested the parts that may be affected.

7. Q: Can radiation protection accessories for X-ray diagnostic equipment be applied for registration combined with the diagnostic equipment?

A: The accessories for radiation protection in the use of X-ray radiation diagnostic equipment, such as radiation protective clothing, radiation protective cap, radiation protective apron, radiation protection collar and medical radiation protective glasses, are used for the protection of human body in radiation diagnosis. Such protection accessories generally have no electrical or physical connection with the X-ray diagnostic equipment. As they are separately regulated as medical devices according to the *Classification Catalogue of Medical Devices*, it is recommended that they should be applied for registration separately, except for those undetachable accessories.

8. Q: What issues should be paid attention to when the service life of software products is determined, including SaMD (Software as a Medical Device) and SiMD (Software in a Medical Device) ?

A: The service life of SaMD is the software life cycle time limit, which is determined by commercial factors and does not need to provide verification materials.

The service life of SiMD is the same as that of its medical device, without the need of reflecting it separately. The dedicated SaMD is considered as SiMD that the service life requirement of software component is the same as the SaMD. It should be reflected in the study data of service life of its medical device.

9. Q: If the proposed product exchanges data with its supporting product (the supporting product is not in the registration application unit) via a non-network cable mode (e.g. Bluetooth, video cable, storage media), does cybersecurity need to be considered?

A: According to the requirements of the *Guidelines for*

Technical Review of Medical Device Cybersecurity, electronic data exchange modes include wireless and wired networks, one-way and two-way data transmission, and real-time and non-real-time remote control and storage media. As the exchange of video data via a non-network cable mode belongs to electronic data exchange, the corresponding requirements of cybersecurity should be considered.

10. Q: Does the standard GB 16174.2 be applicable for the implantable cardiac defibrillator and its similar product?

A: The implantable cardiac defibrillator has the pacing function, which has been fully considered in the standard of YY 0989.6. Furthermore, relevant provisions on the pacing function have been specified in the standard of YY 0989.6. Therefore, the standard of GB 16174.2 does not need to be cited under the condition that the standards of GB 16174.1 and YY 0989.6 have already been applied in the product technical specifications of the implantable cardiac defibrillator and its similar product.

11. Q: What should be paid attention to in the data of disinfection and sterilization for active medical devices that contain many accessories such as patient monitors?

A: For active medical devices containing many accessories, it is recommended to give some information such as the name of the accessories, disinfection/sterilization method, single use/reusable use, sterilization of production enterprises/end-user sterilization, etc., in the structural order of the application form when submitting the disinfection and sterilization data. Sterilization of production enterprises: the sterilization process (methods and parameters) and sterility assurance level (SAL) should be specified, and a sterilization validation report should be provided. End-user sterilization: the recommended sterilization process (methods and parameters) and the determination basis of the recommended sterilization methods should be specified; for products that can withstand twice or multiple sterilizations, the product tolerance study data for the sterilization methods recommended should be provided. If the method used for sterilization is prone to occurrence of residues, the information of residues and handling methods should be specified, and the study data should be provided. End-user disinfection: the recommended disinfection process (methods and parameters) and determination basis of the recommended disinfection method should be specified.

12. Q: If changes take place in the output current of the charger contained in the active product that has been registered and the corresponding labels also change, is it necessary required a change of registration?

A: It should be analyzed whether the changes of the product technical specifications and other contents described in the *Registration Certificate* are involved. If so, a change of registration should be applied. If not, a change of registration should not be required and only relevant work should be done according to the requirements of the enterprise's quality management system (QMS).

13. Q: What should be paid attention to when biocompatibility evaluation is conducted for attachments of the active medical devices (e.g. patient monitor) that contain multiple accessories in contact with human body?

A: Regarding the active medical devices that contain multiple accessories intended to act on human body (including direct and indirect contact), as multiple accessories are involved, more application dossiers should be required. In order to facilitate data review, it is recommended to divide the biocompatibility evaluation of the accessories into the following three categories:

(1) If the biocompatibility evaluation is exempted, it is recommended to submit an explanatory document indicating the absence from the situation specified in "Ⅳ. Reevaluation of biological safety of medical devices (Ⅰ) Manufacturers shall consider biological safety reevaluation under the following circumstances" by referring to the Document No.345 (G.S.Y.J.X. [2007]).

(2) If the biocompatibility evaluation is required, it is recommended to select and evaluate the accessories according to the biological evaluation procedures in the risk management process shown in the system method diagram of GB/T 16886.1.

(3) If the biocompatibility test is required, it is recommended to identify the data or test to be supplemented in the complete risk assessment dataset according to Annex A of GB/T 16886.1.

14. Q: What should be paid attention to when biocompatibility evaluation is conducted for the active medical devices (e.g. patient monitor) that contain multiple accessories in contact with human body?

A: Generally, each functional module (e.g. ECG, body temperature, blood oxygen, noninvasive blood pressure, invasive blood pressure, respiration, EEG, anesthesia) of a patient monitor consists of a number of accessories that are in contact with human body. As the number of accessories applied for registration is large, more application dossiers should be required. In order to facilitate data review, it is recommended to refer to the following requirements:

(1) List the following information in a table according to the structural order of the application form and the classification of the functional modules: names, contact parts, contact time, contact natures and biological evaluation methods (exemption, evaluation and test) of the accessories in contact with human body as well as names and numbers of the corresponding evaluation data.

(2) Clarify the biological test items, test basis, test results, No. of test report, etc. if a biological test is performed.

(3) Explain the reasons for selecting the representative models if representative accessories are selected for tests.

15. Q: If the foot switch contained in the application product is connected with other components through Bluetooth and realizes the remote control function, does cybersecurity need to be considered?

A: The Bluetooth remote control function belongs to electronic data exchange, and risks related to cybersecurity should be considered, and the corresponding materials should be submitted with reference to the *Guidelines for Technical Review of Medical Device Cybersecurity*.

16. Q: Does the standards GB 9706.1 and YY 9706.102 standards be applicable when applying for dental handpiece registration?

A: The lighting power supply methods of the dental handpiece and the connector are divided into three types: with lighting device, light guide type, and non-illuminated type. Products with lighting devices include lighting sources; light-guiding products do not contain lighting sources, but only light-guiding fiber bundles; non-illuminated products contain neither lighting sources nor light-guiding devices.Products with lighting devices should apply GB 9706.1 and YY 9706.102 standards, light-guiding and non-illuminated products do not need to apply GB 9706.1 and YY 9706.102 standards.

17. Q: Can the model of high-voltage generator of registered CT equipment be applied as the same registration unit?

A: If the model of high-voltage generator is added, the performance of the whole machine is essentially equivalent, and it can be used as the same registration unit in principle. Additional models of X-ray combined head of oral cone beam CT equipment can be implemented by reference.

18. Q: When applying for registration of an endoscopic surgical system, what parts are usually included in the product structure and composition?

A: Endoscopic surgical systems are also commonly referred to as "surgical robots". When applying for registration, the product structure and composition usually include a doctor's console, a patient's surgical platform and an image processing platform, and are used in conjunction with 3D laparoscopic endoscopes and surgical instruments. Generally, components or accessories that are not physically or electrically connected to the system are not included in the system registration. Special components or accessories that are physically or electrically connected to the system can be included in the system registration, or separately. For those devices that are commonly used in clinical and connected to the system, such as endoscopic cold light source, high-frequency surgical equipment, etc., usually are not included in the system registration.

19. Q: How to evaluate the residual toxicity of medical devices which are disinfected or sterilized by glutaraldehyde?

A: There are currently no recognized standards or methods for the limit and testing of glutaraldehyde residual toxicity.

According to GB/T 16886.1*Biological evaluation of medical devices - Part 1: Evaluation and testing within a risk management process*, the overall biological evaluation should consider the expected additives, process contaminants and residues. Therefore, if the medical device samples for biological testing have been disinfected or sterilized by glutaraldehyde in accordance with the method prescribed by the administrative counterpart, and the test results meet the requirements of biocompatibility, the residual toxicity of this device is considered acceptable.

In addition to glutaraldehyde, other medical devices residual toxicity processed by chemical disinfectants or sterilants (such as peracetic acid, O-phthalaldehyde, etc.) can also be evaluated in the same way.

20. Q: The composition of active medical device products usually includes a cart, is it necessary to be tested with a cart during the electromagnetic compatibility testing?

A: The electromagnetic compatibility test layout can be divided into floor-mounted equipment and desktop equipment. The two layouts' requirements are different, so the test results may be different. Therefore, if a cart is required in actual use, the electromagnetic compatibility test should include a cart, and the test should be carried out in accordance with the floor-standing equipment; if a cart is not required, the electromagnetic compatibility should be tested in accordance with the desktop equipment. If both conditions are possible in actual use (which means the cart is an optional accessory), the electromagnetic compatibility test should be tested in accordance with both layouts of floor-standing equipment and desktop equipment.

21. Q: Do single-used electronic endoscopes, 3D endoscopes, and capsule endoscopes belong to the *Catalogue of Medical Devices Exempted from Clinical Evaluation*? Are there any other endoscopic medical devices not belonging to the *Catalogue of Medical Devices Exempted from Clinical Evaluation*?

A: The endoscopes described in the *Catalogue of Medical Devices Exempted from Clinical Evaluation* are limited to products of common design, including traditional optical endoscopes, fiber endoscopes and electronic endoscopes. These products are all integrated and reusable designed, expected to be used in conjunction with cold light sources and video cameras/image processors.

Single-used electronic endoscopes (including totally single-used endoscopes and combined endoscopes which concludes a single-used insertion part), 3D endoscopes and capsule endoscopes are not belong to the *Catalogue of Medical Devices Exempted from Clinical Evaluation*. In addition, endoscopes with built-in light sources also don't belong to *Catalogue of Medical Devices Exempted from Clinical Evaluation*.

22. Q: The industry standard of particular medical device recommends that the equipment should work normally within the AC range of 220V ± 22V, while the nominal working voltage of the device is 100-240V, which conflicts with the requirements of the industry standard. Which voltage should be used in the product testing?

A: First of all, the initial consideration of the relevant provision in this standard is to solve the problem whether a device can work normally while meeting the voltage fluctuations that may occur when used in China. Second, the nominal voltage range of the device is only the rated voltage that it claims to be able to support, which is not the same point as the previous one, so there are no contradictions between the two parameters. Therefore, for the situation described in the question, the submission of registration should be accordance with the actual design of the product, which means the nominal voltage range in the "Product Technical Requirements" should be based on the actual design parameter as 100-240V, and the electrical safety and electromagnetic compatibility testing should also be carried out in accordance with the nominal voltage range at 100-240V. While for the testing of the specific provision in industry standard, it should meet the power supply range of 220V ± 22V.

23. Q: Medical device software adds new clinical functions, and the administrative counterpart considers that the software update is a minor software update, so the software release version remains unchanged, is it allowed?

A: Changes in clinical functions should be considered as a major software update. When the naming rules for software versions prescribed by the administrative counterpart cannot clearly distinguish major software updates from minor software updates, it should follow the principle of higher risk adoption, consider it as a major software update. For example, the software version naming convention is X.Y.Z, where X represents major software updates, Y represents that cannot distinguish between major and minor software updates, and Z represents minor software updates, then the software release version should be X.Y.

24. Q: The testing result of an active medical device reflects a large tolerance in the particular parameter, and it does not meet the relevant requirements, is it possible to change the nominal value of this parameter according to the testing result, so that the tolerance of this parameter could meet the requirements?

A: The nominal value of the product is determined based on the product requirements, and the tolerance is comprehensively considered based on the deviation of the production process and test equipment. These two data of the parameter belong to the design characteristics of the product and cannot be modified simply based on the inspection report data. If the nominal value and tolerance of the parameter need to be modified, the administrative counterpart should first consider whether this will have influence on the product design and quality management system. If the changes are involved, the design input of relevant parameters should be modified, and additional tests should be carried on the samples which are produced after the design change.

25. Q: For imported products, the indication for use of the main unit and its accessories are inconsistent while approved by the country (origin) where the applicant or filling entity is registered or the manufacture is carried out. When submitted in China as a whole system, is it possible to integrate the indication for use of the two parts?

A: First thing to consider is determination that whether the main unit and its accessory could be submitted together as a whole registration, according to the *Guidance for the Division of Medical Device Registration Units*.

If so, the indication for use which submitted in the registration could integrate its original indications for the main unit and accessories.

When the indication for use of the two parts is inconsistent, the content that jointly included by the two parts should be selected. It is also needed to consider the reference of the approved similar products, but not exceed the indication for use which approved by the country (origin) where the applicant or filling entity is registered or the manufacture is carried out.

26. Q: For the animal test of ultrasound soft tissue surgical device, if there are multiple typical models of ultrasound surgical instruments, how to decide the test sample of animal individuals and vessel processing in the animal testing?

A: For products which have multiple ultrasound surgical instruments, the typical ultrasound surgical instruments could be selected according to the requirements of "X. Animal testing (4) Animal testing requirements" from the *Guidance of Technical Review for Ultrasound Soft Tissue Surgical Device*. If it is considered that there are multiple typical models of ultrasound surgical instruments, different typical model should be evaluated independently, and the test sample of vessel processing should be calculated independently.

For the acute animal test, the effect of multiple processing on the normal physiological state of the test animal should be considered, in order to ensure that the blood vessel and soft tissue are in a normal physiological state during each following processing procedure. For the chronic animal test, it is recommended not to test multiple ultrasound surgical instruments on the same animal, in case of the problems that unexpected situation emerges however cannot be distinguishably analyzed.

27. Q: For the electromagnetic compatibility test of ultrasound soft tissue surgical device, is it possible to choose one typical model ultrasound surgical instrument?

A: Common ultrasound surgical instruments (without transducer) only conduct sound energy, not electric energy, which theoretically has no effect on electromagnetic compatibility performance. However, it is necessary that the test to be carried out accompany with the ultrasound surgical instruments.

In order to accomplish some functions such as identification for single-using or collection of working parameters, some ultrasound surgical instruments have a chip (or RFID) which needs to be powered in it, therefore it may affect the electromagnetic compatibility performance.

It is necessary to consider the difference of multiple models of ultrasound surgical instruments, and select a typical model for testing. For ultrasound surgical instruments without chips, which do not conduct electrical signals or electrical energy, one typical model could be selected for testing.

28. Q: For the microwave ablation equipment and ablation needles, is it possible to be registered separately? Is it necessary to make limitation for the cooperation use?

A: The ablation equipment and ablation needles could be submitted registration totally, or separately.

The matching requirements of the microwave generator, cables and ablation needles are highly recommended. Changing the accompany patterns informally will seriously affect the safety and efficacy of the microwave output. Therefore, the research, development, production and use must be coordinated between the specified generator and accessories.

For the microwave ablation equipment and ablation needles which are submitted separately, the use restrictions of cooperation must be clearly defined. The microwave generator submitted separately should declare the cooperation use of the microwave needles which are approved in the indication for use. The microwave needles submitted separately should declare the model and software version of the cooperation generator.

29. Q: What types of endoscopic power surgical equipment are included? How to determine the main performance parameters of various products?

A: Endoscopic power surgical equipment refers to a product that uses a power-driven device to provide mechanical force for surgical instruments to mince or cut tissues during endoscopic surgery. Endoscopic power surgical equipment can be divided into different types according to the purpose of shaving, grinding or drilling which realized by the surgical instruments. For example, equipment for soft tissue shaving, equipment for bone tissue grinding/drilling, and devices with both functions above.

The main performance parameters of the product should be determined with reference to the corresponding national standards and industry standards, combined with clinical requirements and the technical characteristics of the product itself. Among them, the equipment used for shaving should meet the requirements of the industry standard YY/T 0955 *Medical Endoscopes: Endoscope surgical equipment - Shaver*, and the equipment used for other purposes (such as grinding or drilling) can refer to this standard and combining the characteristics of the product.

30. Q: The high-frequency and ultrasound integrated surgical equipment can not only output high-frequency or ultrasound energy separately, but also output two kinds of energy at the same time. How to determine the test mode during electromagnetic compatibility test?

A: For the emission test, according to GB 4824 *Industrial, scientific and medical equipment-Radio-frequency disturbance characteristics-Limits and methods for measurement*, the ultrasound surgical equipment should be divided into Group 1, and the high-frequency surgical equipment should be Group 2, but according to GB 9706.4/GB 9706.202 *Medical electrical equipment-Part 2-2: Particular requirements for the basic safety and essential performance of high frequency surgical equipment and high frequency surgical accessories*, high frequency surgical equipment should comply with group 1 when it is switched on and in an idle state with the HF output not energized. Therefore, the emissions test of integrated surgical equipment should be tested in the worst case (at least the maximum ultrasound output mode should be included), and the test should be classified as Group 1 Class A.

For the immunity test, the standby mode, ultrasound output mode, high frequency output mode and dual output mode should be selected respectively, and the test should be carried out under the worst case.

31. Q: Active surgical equipment includes a variety of surgical instruments. In order to provide different types and quantities of surgical instruments for the requirement of medical facilities, is it possible that surgical instruments be declared in the form of "optional accessories"?

A: If a certain part of the product composition of a medical device is necessary to achieve its intended use and basic function, it cannot be considered as an "optional accessory". If the surgical device is expected to be optional and users could choose different models to achieve different functions, it can be submitted registration in the form of "optional accessories". Purchasing one or part of the surgical instruments separately or not does not affect the safety and efficacy of the overall use of the product.

Whether the surgical instrument is declared in the form of "optional accessories" or not, the technical review requirements are the same, and all the instruments need to be declared in the product structure and composition.

Chapter 2

Common technical issues of non-active medical device

32. Q: For flexible corneal contact lens products, what factors should be considered when selecting or changing the primary packaging materials?

A: Since the risk of free substances in the primary packaging materials of soft corneal contact lens products being extracted by the solution, which may affect the performance and safety of the contact lens, attention should be paid when selecting or changing the primary packaging materials:

(1) The performance of the primary packaging materials should be verified, including physical and chemical properties, and biological evaluation (e.g.leachables analysis, biological testing, etc.).

(2) Sterilization suitability research and sterilization confirmation for primary packaging materials.

(3) It is recommended to conduct product stability verification in accordance with GB/T 11417.8 *Ophthalmic optics—Contact lenses—Part 8: Determination of shelf-life*, including lens performance, packaging integrity, sterility, etc. It is recommended to conduct research on the performance of the preservation solution.

(4) Carry out transportation stability verification on primary packaging materials.

(5) If there are two or more kinds of primary packaging, the final product with different primary packaging should be tested for full performance and biological evaluation. Full performance includes all design verification performance and all performance indicators in technical requirements.

(6) If the primary packaging material that has never been used

in similar products is used, it is recommended to evaluate and verify the leachate that may be contained in the preservation solution in the stability test.

33. Q: Contact lens care products such as those claiming to be suitable for silicone hydrogel lenses, what information and precautions need to be submitted?

A: According to YY 0719.5*Ophthalmic optics—Contact lens care products—Part 5: Determination of physical compatibility of contact lens care products with contact lenses*, the compatibility test between care products and silicone hydrogel lenses should be conducted separately. Administrative counterparts should select a representative silicone hydrogel lenses that have been marketed for research and submit validation information. Product technical requirements document should be clearly detected the use of silicone hydrogel lenses, and attached to the self-test report issued by administrative counterparts or the inspection report commissioned by a qualified medical device inspection agency as supporting information. If the above information is not submitted, the scope of application should be expressly not applicable to silicone hydrogel lenses.

34. Q: For injectable cross-linked sodium hyaluronate gel products, if the pre-filled syringe is a purchased product with a registration certificate, is it necessary to develop the relevant performance requirements in the product technical requirements document?

A: In view of the fact that the prefilled syringe not only serves as the inner packaging container of the device, but also has the function of injection, so regardless of whether they have obtained the qualification of pharmaceutical packaging materials or medical device registration certificates, it is necessary to set functional and safety indicators and test methods related to them in the product technical requirements document from the perspective of finished products, which can be objectively determined, such as pushing force, appearance of syringe, scale, performance of conical joint (for non-conical joint, it is required that the cooperation between syringe and injection needle has no leakage), effective capacity (or filling capacity), body tightness (no gel leakage at the piston or test with water), fit between the piston and the outer casing (the core rod does not move due to gravity when it is kept vertical), etc.For specific performance indicators and test methods, please refer to GB 15810 *Sterile syringe for single use* or relevant national/industry standards.

35. Q: If a soft hydrophilic contact lens is declared as ionic or non-ionic, how to submit relevant research information?

A: If the administrative counterpart claims that the soft hydrophilic contact lens is ionic or non-ionic, it should be determined according to the definition of ionic and non-ionic in GB/T 11417.1*Ophthalmic optics—Contact lenses—Part 1: Vocabulary, classification system and recommendations for labeling specifications.* Firstly, the nature of each monomer in the product formulation needs to be clarified, such as ionic, non-ionic, etc., followed by calculating the content of ionic monomer (expressed in molar fraction), and finally making a conclusion based on the relevant requirements of GB/T 11417.1*Ophthalmic optics— Contact lenses—Part 1: Vocabulary, classification system and recommendations for labeling specifications*, and specifying the soft hydrophilic contact lens as ionic or non-ionic in the appendix of the product technical requirements.

36. Q: For intravascular catheters, under what circumstances is it necessary to provide research data on flow rate and to develop it in the product technical requirements?

A: (1) If there is a nominal flow rate in the IFU/labels or other information of the intravascular catheter, relevant research data on the flow rate should be provided.

(2) For catheters that infuse drugs into the body, such as central venous catheters, the flow rate should be specified and the flow rate requirements should be developed in the technical requirements document.

(3) Because the perfusion pressure in the flow/velocity detection method in Appendix E of YY0285.1 *Intravascular catheters— Sterile and single-use catheters—Part 1: General requirements* is about 10kPa. The flow requirements in this standard do not apply to products with nominal flow rates greater than 10kPa perfusion pressure. For products with a perfusion pressure exceeding 10kPa, the flow requirements may not be formulated in the product technical requirements document, but the corresponding verification data need to be provided in the research data.

37. Q: For intravascular angiography catheters, under what circumstances should power injection be considered for the request?For those that need to consider the power injection requirements, what should be paid attention to in product registration?

A: (1) For contrast catheter products using high-pressure injection devices for injection, the technical requirements document and IFU (labeling) to mark the maximum burst pressure information, while the power injection requirements in accordance with YY0285.1*Intravascular catheters—Sterile and single-use catheters—Part 1: General requirements*.

(2) For contrast catheter products using a ring handle syringe to inject contrast media, power injection requirements may not be developed. It is appropriate to specify the following warning in the instruction manual: Do not use high-pressure injection devices to inject contrast media.

(3) For other catheters with angiographic functions in the scope of application, it is appropriate to refer to the above requirements.

38. Q: What considerations need to be taken when the biological test report of the similar device that has been marketed by the administrative counterpart is used to replace the biological test report of the declared product?

A: (1) The administrative counterpart needs to confirm the chemical composition of the tested products and the declared products in the test report, the chemical composition of materials, the proportion of each constituent material, the physical structure of the product, the surface characteristics, the production process, the sterilization method, the raw material suppliers and technical specifications, Any factors that may affect biological risks, such as inner packaging materials (if applicable, mainly involving liquid products and wet storage products), are completely consistent, and relevant declarations are provided.

(2) If there is inconsistency between the test product and the declared product in the factors listed above that may affect the biological risk, sufficient reasons and evidence should be provided to support the submitted test report for the declared product, and if necessary, supplement the corresponding biological evaluation data, such as leachable analysis and toxicological risk assessment data, supplementary tests of related biological test items, etc.

(3) The biological test report of similar products is only used to replace the test report of the declared product as part of the biological evaluation, not to replace the overall biological evaluation report of the declared product.

39. Q: What is the selection principle of quantitative evaluation and qualitative evaluation of cytotoxicity evaluation? Which evaluation method is preferred?

A: The quantitative evaluation of cytotoxicity can objectively measure the number of cells, total protein, enzyme release, living dye release, living dye reduction or other measurable parameters. It is not easy to be affected by the subjective factors of the experimenter. It has relatively high sensitivity and clear judgment limit. At present, MTT quantitative method is widely used in China. Relatively speaking, the qualitative evaluation of cytotoxicity has more subjectivity and is more suitable for screening. In addition, the results of qualitative evaluation and quantitative evaluation are inconsistent in the actual test (for example, substances exist in the extract of the sample that cause great changes in the absorbance of the culture medium, etc.). Therefore, it is recommended to take the quantitative evaluation method as the basic method. At the same time, it is necessary to examine the cell morphology under microscope and report the results, supplemented by qualitative evaluation if necessary.

40. Q: Is it necessary that the virus inactivation process of animal derived medical devices must be verified in the laboratory to evaluate the virus inactivation effect?

A: According to the *Guidelines for Technical Review of Animal Origin Medical Device Registration*, when applying for the product registration of animal origin, the research data submitted should include the description of the process of inactivating and removing viruses and / or infectious factors in the production process and the effectiveness verification data or relevant materials. Different animal sources, production processes and applicable products have different risks. The research data of virus inactivation effect can be obtained through laboratory verification or from the supplier of animal derived materials. For products with mature raw material application, if they adopt mature virus inactivation process and have appropriate literature, the virus inactivation effect can also be evaluated through literature or historical data. If the submitted verification data is not based on the data obtained from the verification of the declared product itself, it is necessary to analyze and demonstrate the applicability.

41. Q: GB/T 16886.1 *Biological evaluation of medical devices—Part 1: Evaluation and testing within a risk management process* **and** *Notice on guidelines for biological evaluation and review of medical devices* **(CFDA[2007]No. 345) all mention exemption from biological test. How can surgical devices be exempted from biological test?**

A: Based on the current cognitive level, if the materials in direct or indirect contact with patients in surgical instruments are only composed of metal materials, they are verified to meet the relevant national, industrial and international standards for metal materials for surgical implants or materials for surgical instruments, as well as the brand specified in the relevant product standards, The biological test can be exempted when the verification data of the chemical composition of the material is provided (if it is demonstrated that the production process does not affect the chemical composition of the material, it can be submitted in the form of raw material bill).

42. Q: If the cross-linked sodium hyaluronate gel product for injection contains purchased injection needle accessories with registration certificate, what performance studies should be carried out for the accessories?

A: For cross-linked sodium hyaluronate gel products for injection, if it contains purchased injection needle accessories with registration certificate, quality control standards, test reports and supporting documents (such as medical device registration certificates, etc.) of purchased injection needles should be submitted.

（1）If the purchased injection needle is sterilized by ethylene oxide（EO）, the administrative counterpart should provide information（such as supplier inspection report or incoming inspection report, etc.）to prove that the EO residual risk of injection needle has been controlled. In view of the fact that EO residue risk is controlled when entering the factory, and the risk decreases with the time after entering the factory, if new EO risk is not introduced in the production process, EO residue requirements may not be formulated in the product technical requirements of crosslinked sodium hyaluronate gel for injection.

（2）If the injection needle has not obtained the registration certificate, the relevant verification data of the injection needle should be provided in the research data. The administrative counterpart is primarily responsible for the safety and effectiveness of purchased accessories. Therefore, the performance requirements and testing methods of injection needles should be formulated in the product technical requirements document with reference to GB 15811 *Sterile hypodermic needles for single use*, and an inspection report should be provided.

43. Q: For passive vascular implant devices containing delivery systems or accessories, do the implanted components and delivery systems or accessories need to be biologically evaluated separately?

A: For passive vascular implantable medical devices containing delivery systems or accessories, such as implantable stents and occluders pre-installed on the delivery systems, it is expected that the parts that remain in the human body for the long term are significantly different from their delivery systems or accessories in terms of contact properties and/or contact time with the human body. When registering this kind of products, it is advisable to carry out biological evaluation on the components and delivery systems or accessories that are expected to remain in the human body for the long term. Thermal test can be combined.

44. Q: What should be paid attention to when comparing the mechanical properties of hernia repair patches exempted from clinical evaluation with products registered in China in *Catalogue of Medical Devices Exempted from Clinical Evaluation*?

A: For hernia repair meshes exempted from clinical evaluation, when the tensile strength, tensile elongation and bursting strength meet the clinical standards, no comparison is required. If the tensile elongation is different from the clinical acceptance standard, it is necessary to conduct a comparative study with the products registered in China to demonstrate that the risk is acceptable. The weight per unit area, pore size, porosity / mesh density of the declared product is generally equivalent to the products registered in China in *Catalogue of Medical Devices Exempted from Clinical Evaluation*. The tear strength (only applicable to trouser patch), suture strength, connection strength, etc., of the declared product should be no worse than similar products already on the market.

45. Q: What should be paid attention to when developing the tensile strength and elongation performance index of hernia repair patch?

A: (1) If the tensile strength of the patch is different due to material design, weaving process and other reasons, the longitudinal and transverse tensile strength should be formulated respectively.

(2) It is suggested to establish the tensile elongation under the maximum abdominal wall tension that human physiological conditions may be subjected to. The acceptance standard of tensile elongation should be formulated by combining the elongation of natural abdominal wall of human body and the measured data of hernia patch. If the tensile elongation of the patch is different due to material design, weaving process and other reasons, the longitudinal and transverse tensile elongation should be formulated respectively.

46. Q: Why is heat treatment required after laser selective melting metal materials for additive manufacturing dental restorations, and what research data are required?

A: Since the laser selective melting of metal materials for dental prosthetics may generate thermal stress, tissue stress and residual stress during the printing and forming process, it is easy to cause warpage deformation and cracks of the final product, resulting in low plasticity of the final product, so heat treatment is required. The general heat treatment process includes tempering, annealing, etc. For the research of heat treatment process, it is generally necessary to clarify the heat treatment process method and heat treatment process parameters of the product, evaluate and verify the suitability of the heat treatment method, and provide the basis for determining the heat treatment process parameters (such as heating time, holding temperature, holding time, etc.), and demonstrate the clinical acceptability of heat treatment results.

47. Q: What should be included in non-clinical research of unicompartmental knee joint prostheses?

A: Unicompartmental knee prostheses are used to replace the femoral and tibial articular surfaces of the medial or lateral compartment of the knee, usually including a femoral component and a tibial component, where the tibial component consists of a tibial insert and a tibial tray. When designing and developing such products, administrative counterparts can refer to YY 0502 *Joint replacement implants— Knee joint prostheses*, YY/T 0919 *Non-active surgical implants—Joint replacement implants—Specific requirements for knee-joint replacement implants*, YY/T 0924 *Implant for surgery Components for partial and total knee joint prostheses* series of standards, etc. Non-clinical research of products should at least include the following:

(1) Related research data on articular surface design.

(2) The research on mechanical properties generally includes fatigue properties of femoral components, fatigue properties of tibial trays, and joint wear properties.

(3) Biological evaluation data of the product.

(4) The sterilization verification confirmation data of the product.

(5) Verification data of the shelf life of the product.

48. Q: What are the general contents of the mechanical properties of metal cannulate bone screws?

A: The scope of application of metal cannulate bone screws is generally used for the internal fixation of limb fractures. It is divided into two situations: used alone or used in conjunction with metal bone plates, usually, the mechanical properties need to be studied. Combined with the product characteristics and intended use, the mechanical properties study should at least evaluate the screw's maximum torque and fracture torsion angle, axial pull-out performance, screw-in torque and screw-out torque performance. If the screw also has self-tapping ability, its self-tapping performance should also be evaluated. For screw-in torque and screw-out torque performance, in addition to avoiding screw breakage during product design, administrative counterparts should also ensure that doctor can easily screw in and out. Therefore, attention should be paid to the screw-in torque and screw-out torque should not be too large.

49. Q: What does the research on the mechanical properties of self-stabilizing intervertebral body cages generally include?

A: Self-stabilizing intervertebral body cages are generally composed of intervertebral body cages, metal plates and screws. Because they do not require additional spinal internal fixation devices, they are often called self-stabilizing intervertebral body cages. It is mostly used for interbody fusion in the cervical spine. When evaluating the mechanical properties of the self-stabilizing interbody cage, it is necessary to consider the performance of the interbody cage itself, such as compression performance, compression shear performance, torsional performance, subsidence, etc. The performance of metal plates used to replace the function of spinal internal fixation devices should be considered, such as bending performance, torsion performance, etc. The long-term stability of the connection structure and system structure of the metal plate and the cage, the torsional performance and fixation strength of the screw, etc., should also be considered. The administrative counterpart can carry out relevant experiments by simulating the clinical use method based on the structural characteristics of the product.

50. Q: What should be considered in the worst-case selection of test samples when performing system performance tests for the surgical fixation of the thoracic lumbar spinal skeletal system for posterior implantation?

A: The performance test of the surgical fixation of the thoracic lumbar spinal skeletal system for posterior implantation generally includes system compression test, system tension test, and system torsion test. When selecting the worst case sample for system test, factors such as product design type, size specification, assembly situation and locking mechanism between components should be considered. Different performance tests have different stress patterns, and the worst-case samples for each test may be different. In general, the failure of the sample in the system dynamic fatigue test may occur in addition to the fracture of the locking screw thread root, and the rod failure may also occur. Therefore, to determine the worst case of the test sample, the influence of the characteristics of the rod (such as material, specification, design type, surface treatment method), the locking method between the components and the assembly situation on the system performance should be comprehensively considered. Component risks that cannot be reflected in systematic tests can be evaluated through component tests to comprehensively demonstrate the clinical acceptability of the test results.

51. Q: What key points should be considered in the design of coating for joint prostheses?

A: The coating for joint prosthesis is mainly used to improve the adhesion between bone tissue and joint prostheses fixed without bone cement, so the design of the coating determines the expected osseointegration effect. Coating parameters that should usually be specified include at least coating porosity, coating thickness, coating pore intercept, coating surface roughness (if applicable), etc. The rationality of coating parameter design can be based on reference to similar marketed products or existing long-term clinical application data to support the evidence that the coating design can achieve stable fixation of the prosthesis. In the case of new coating materials, new coating processes, or new coating parameter designs, a decision can be made as to whether animal testing studies are required to demonstrate the effectiveness of the coating.

52. Q: What issues should be paid attention to when registering a shoulder prostheses product?

A: Shoulder prostheses generally include glenoid components and humeral components. Common shoulder prostheses products include positive shoulder prostheses and reverse shoulder prostheses. If the same component has the same material and different components are used together as a whole, positive shoulder prostheses and reverse shoulder prostheses with similar structural composition can be registered and declared together. The performance evaluation of shoulder prostheses should at least consider the mechanical strength of each component, the connection stability between components, the wear performance of the articular surface, and the range of motion of the joint. If the component is coated, the performance of the coating should also be considered.

53. Q: What aspects should generally be considered for in vitro degradation testing of degradable implants for osteosynthesis?

A: For degradable implants for osteosynthesis, in order to ensure that it can provide strong internal fixation for damaged bone tissue, combined with the fracture healing period, its ability to provide initial stability needs to be evaluated. Therefore, in vitro research on the degradation properties of degradable implants for osteosynthesis are generally required. The research should at least include the degradation rate of the product, the change of the mechanical properties with the time during the degradation process, the degradation products of the product and the degradation cycle of the product. The end point of the observation time of the product degradation performance test should be considered to reach the steady state of degradation or until the product is completely degraded.

54. Q: What aspects should be paid attention to when evaluating the deformation resistance of metal acetabular shells in hip joint prostheses?

A: For the test method for evaluating the deformation resistance of metal acetabular shells, please refer to YY/T 0809.12 *Implants for surgery— Partial and total hip joint prostheses— Part 12: Deformation test method for Acetabular shells*. The residual difference in the initial diameter obtained by the test method described in this standard is greater than 2% of the obtained deformation. This 2% is not an acceptable standard for the deformation resistance of the acetabular cup, but indicates that the product is plastically deformed, and should be stop testing this specimen and select a new specimen to retest. When evaluating the anti-deformation performance of the acetabular shell, the administrative counterpart should provide an acceptable basis for the test results, and should consider the anti-deformation ability of the acetabular shell itself and the impact on the acetabular lining in combination with the actual clinical application of the product. Since the metal acetabular shell is expected to be used in conjunction with the acetabular lining, in addition to the deformation of the acetabular shell itself, the deformation after the assembly of the acetabular shell and the lining should also be considered.

55. Q: How to choose the worst-case sample for mechanical performance of intervertebral body cages?

A: In the study of mechanical properties of intervertebral body cages, the worst-case samples should usually be selected for testing.

Cages for cervical spine and cages for thoracic and lumbar spine should be selected as worst-case samples due to different forces. The influence of factors such as bone graft area size, side hole size, inclination angle, length, width and height of different types of cages on the mechanical properties of the product should be considered. At the same time, the stress conditions of different mechanical properties are different, and the selected worst-case samples may also be different. Combined with the dynamic and static mechanical performance test methods and loading methods, finite element analysis methods can be used to determine the worst-case samples of cages for cervical spine and cages for thoracic and lumbar spine.

56. Q: Is it necessary to consider the impact of product batches on product performance when conducting research on the performance of medical device products?

A: For most medical devices (non-in vitro diagnostic reagents), the stability and validity period of various properties of the product usually depend on the raw materials used in the product and the aging mechanism of the materials, such as thermal aging, photoaging, etc. As long as the raw material properties, production process and packaging materials of the product remain stable, in principle, the differences between batches should not affect the performance stability and validity period of the product. Therefore, in general, batches do not need to be considered when conducting performance studies. If the product has special characteristics, such as containing biologically active substances, the impact of batch-to-batch variation on product performance can be considered.

57. Q: In the shelf life study of passive medical devices, if real-time stability verification is carried out, how should the verification temperature be considered?

A: Theoretically, the temperature of the real-time stability study of the product is generally the same as the storage temperature. If some products have special regulations, the relevant regulations will be implemented first. For example, GB/T 11417.8 *Ophthalmic optics—Contact lenses—Part 8: Determination of shelf-life*, the standard clearly stipulates that the temperature used in the stability study of contact lens products is 25. However, for general medical devices stored at room temperature, if there are no special regulations, in principle, the real-time stability verification temperature is not mandatory to be performed at 25°C ± 2°C, and corresponding research data can be provided according to product characteristics. For medical devices with special requirements for storage temperature, verification research should be carried out according to the specified temperature.

58. Q: How to evaluate the allogeneic medical device virus inactivation study?

A: Allogeneic medical devices, that is, medical devices made from human tissues, such as allogeneic bone and allogeneic tendon, the risks of biological safety such as product viruses or infectious factors need to be considered. Therefore, it is necessary to verify the effectiveness of the virus inactivation process of the product. For some common virus inactivation processes, such as organic solvents, radiation irradiation, strong acid and alkali, etc., the process and method are relatively mature, and there are many literature evidences that can be referred to. For products with relatively mature raw material applications, the administrative counterpart can evaluate the effect of virus inactivation process through literature or historical data, and can also evaluate virus inactivation effect through virus inactivation process verification test.

59. Q: How can absorbable medical device products be exempted from in vivo metabolism studies?

A: Because the raw materials of absorbable medical device products can be absorbed by the human body, their metabolism in the body may pose safety risks, and it is necessary to pay attention to their metabolism in the human body. However, for most mature materials, such as sodium hyaluronate, animal collagen, chitosan, starch, polylactic acid, etc., there are many relevant research literatures, and their metabolic pathways are relatively fixed. Metabolic pathways have less impact and generally do not change significantly. Therefore, for the products prepared from the above-mentioned mature materials, the administrative counterpart may not provide the in vivo metabolism research data of the product, but can verify the safety of the product by providing existing literature data as support, or through biocompatibility evaluation. If the product uses a new absorbable material and there is a lack of relevant research data on the in vivo metabolism of the material, an in vivo metabolism study of the product is required.

60. Q: Should the performance index of the product material be specified in the product technical requirement document?

A: According to the requirements of the *Administrative Measures for the Registration and Filing of Medical Devices*, the performance indicators in the product technical requirements document mainly refer to the functional and safety indicators of the finished medical device that can be objectively judged. Therefore, the material properties of general products are not included in the performance indicators of product technical requirements documents, including but not limited to the chemical composition, microstructure and internal quality of metal product materials, Infrared spectrum of polymer product materials, chemical composition, impurity element content, thermal conductivity, and crystal phase content of ceramic product materials. For material characterization information that is indeed related to product safety, it can be stated in the form of an appendix in the technical requirements document.

61. Q: How to submit an application for changes in the contents of IFU that are not within the scope of change registration?

A: For changes in the contents of IFU that do not fall within the scope of change registration, the administrative counterpart may submit an application for notification on IFU change. According to the provisions of Article 3 of the *Operating standard for IFU change notification review of medical devices*, if the IFU of a registered medical device has changed other than the items specified in the registration certificate and its attachments, which does not belong to the scope of change registration, it can be changed after review and approval. Therefore, if the content of IFU that does not fall within the scope of change registration has changed, when submitting the application for notification on IFU change, if it is deemed necessary to submit corresponding evidence, the administrative counterpart must submit the supporting research data of the changed content together. The reviewers need to combine the research data to comprehensively review whether changes are allowed. If the review believes that it does not fall within the scope of notification on IFU change, they need to explain the reasons to the administrative counterpart.

62. Q: If an orthopaedic medical device has passed the equivalence test to prove that it is equivalent to a marketed product, is it necessary to select the worst-case for performance research?

A: The performance research data provided by the administrative counterpart should always focus on the declared product, and consider the impact of key dimensions, structural design and other factors on product performance. For different performance studies, the worst-case for each performance was selected to conduct the corresponding test, and the clinical acceptability of the test results should be evaluated. In assessing the clinical acceptability of test results, the means of demonstrating equivalence to marketed products through equivalence testing may be considered. Even if the declared product and the marketed product have the same scope of application, indications, and expected usage (for example, there is a previous generation product, and the declared product only has a certain difference in product structure compared with it), it should be based on the above in principle.

63. Q: What aspects should be considered in the matching of laser selective melting metal powder and printing parameters for additive manufacturing dental restoration?

A: The matching of metal powder for additive manufacturing and printing parameters mainly involves the production process of metal powder and the key process parameters of printing equipment. Regarding the production process of metal powder, the key process principle and selection basis should be explained (such as electrode induction melting gas atomization, plasma inert gas atomization, vacuum induction melting gas atomization, plasma rotating electrode atomization, etc.), identify key process parameters (such as gas pressure, flow rate and temperature, inner diameter and spray angle of gas atomizing nozzle, pressure and oxygen content in gas atomizing tower, current and speed of rotary electrode atomization process, etc.), and submit relevant research data. Regarding the matching with the key process parameters of the printing equipment, process parameters such as laser power, spot diameter, scanning speed, scanning distance, powder thickness, printing direction, atmosphere protection, support structure, and forming chamber temperature should be considered, and relevant research data should be submitted.

64. Q: If an orthopaedic medical device is made of materials that are acceptable for clinical use as described in Appendix B of YY 0341.1 *Non-active surgical implants— Osteosynthesis and spinal implants—Part 1: Particular requirements for osteosynthesis implants,* **can the biological evaluation data be submitted in the form of exemption from biological evaluation when submitting the product registration?**

A: The biological evaluation data in the product registration cannot be submitted by exempting biological evaluation. The administrative counterpart can prove that the declared product has the same biocompatibility with the marketed product through equivalence comparison, so as to determine the reduction or exemption of the biological test of the declared product. For materials that meet the requirements in Appendix B of YY 0341.1 *Non-active surgical implants—Osteosynthesis and spinal implants—Part 1: Particular requirements for osteosynthesis implants,* biological evaluation is still required by means of equivalence comparison. At the same time, the influence on the biocompatibility of the product by the difference between the structure and shape of the raw material, the structural characteristics of the product, and the production process and the listed product is considered. Taking the production process as an example, the production and processing of products usually introduces new harmful substances (such as residues of sterilants, processing aids, mold release agents, etc.). Therefore, it should be evaluated whether the production and processing process (processing process, sterilization process, packaging, etc.) of the declared product introduces new and same risks. If after evaluation, the declared product does not introduce new biological risks, the biological test can be exempted.

65. Q: How to evaluate the degradation performance of resorbable bone implant products?

A: In general, resorbable bone implant products should be carried out to study the degradation performance of the product, and attention should be paid to the matching of the degradation process with bone growth. The product should be designed in such a way that the initial stability of the product can be maintained for a period of time at the beginning of degradation. For products that need to provide a certain mechanical strength, such as absorbable interface screws, the product should have a certain mechanical strength in the early stage of degradation. Therefore, when conducting product degradation performance studies, the rate of product degradation is of concern. In combination with the time required for clinical bone growth, evaluate the mechanical property changes of the product during the degradation process to ensure that the mechanical strength of the product at the initial stage of degradation can meet clinical needs. At the same time, the degradation rate of the product is ensured to match the rate of bone growth. It is recommended that the administrative counterpart combined with the product material characteristics, structural design and clinical intended use for a comprehensive evaluation, can provide relevant supporting basis through literature research, the same species of product comparison.

66. Q: Is it necessary that the meniscal component thickness of a unicompartmental knee joint prosthesis made of conventional UHMWPE must be at least 6mm?

A: In principle, the meniscal component made of conventional UHMWPE should have a thickness of at least 6mm in the load-bearing area when used with tibial tray. If the product design cannot meet the thickness, should provide product design basis and reasonable justification, and prove that the design can ensure that the product meets the clinical safety and effectiveness, and provide the appropriate supporting basis. If the product is compared with the same variety of products have already been on the market, it should provide the comparison between the declared product and the same variety of products in terms of structural design, key dimensions and mechanical properties, etc. Combined with the clinical application of the same variety of products, a comprehensive evaluation is conducted. Relevant supporting evidence can be provided by retrieving clinical literature data and adverse event data of the same product variety.

67. Q: For orthopaedic implant products made of conventional UHMWPE materials, can the accelerated aging test in the standard YY/T 0772.3 *Implants for surgery Ultra-high-molecular-weight polyethylene Part 3*: *Accelerated ageing methods* and the accelerated aging test in the product stability study be substituted for each other?

A: For orthopaedic implant products made of conventional UHMWPE materials, the administrative counterpart should evaluate the stability (such as oxidation index and mechanical properties before and after aging) and morphology of conventional UHMWPE materials with reference to the methods in the standard YY/T 0772. 3 *Implants for surgery Ultra-high-molecular-weight polyethylene Part 3: Accelerated ageing methods,* YY/T 0772.4 *Implants for surgery Ultra-high-molecular-weight polyethylene Part 4: Oxidation index measurement method,* YY/T 0772.5 *Implants for surgery Ultra-high-molecular-weight polyethylene Part 5: Morphology assessment method* in the research data. The accelerated aging method in the standard cannot simulate the relationship between the test conditions and the real-time storage aging of the product. Therefore, it is not equivalent to a product stability study. The test conditions for the accelerated aging test in product stability studies are based on the assumption that the chemical reactions involved in material deterioration follow the Arrhenius function, which can be inferred from the aging of the material under normal storage conditions of the product. Therefore, the stability of the product (including shelf life) study should refer to the *Guidelines for Stability Studies of Passive Implantable Medical Devices* and submit research data on real-time stability or accelerated stability studies of the product.

68. Q: What items does the suitability of needles and injection pens need to be verified?

A: Relevant verification data should be provided for the application of the product in conjunction with the injection pen, and the performance indicators generally include ease of assembly/ disassembly, needle dose accuracy, unscrewing torque of the needle, etc. The needle is attached to the pen by applying the prescribed torque, the integrity of the clinically relevant fluid pathway is confirmed by a dose accuracy test, and the removal torque of the needle hub is measured and recorded. In addition, when submitting the verification data for the functional suitability of the declared product and the injection pen used in conjunction with it, a reasonable explanation should be provided for the number of products to be verified, and parameters such as confidence and reliability should be specified.

69. Q: How to design the clearance test conditions for haemodialyzer devices?

A: The clearance rate is the main functional parameter of the hemodialyzer and a key indicator for evaluating the quality of the dialyzer. The test conditions for clearance rate should be clear, and the clearance rate test should cover the range of blood flow rate and dialysate flow rate specified by the administrative counterpart. According to YY 0053 *Hemodialysis and relevant therapies—Haemodialysers, haemodiafilters, haemofilters and haemoconcentrators*, in the clearance test of haemodialyzer products, the flow rate of blood and dialysate should cover the range specified by the administrative counterpart. In the test, the dialysate flow rate generally selects the lowest and highest points, which correspond to all the blood flow rates specified in the IFU.

70. Q: What leachables does the hemoditoxifier need to control?

A: First of all, the applicant should strictly restrict the use of high-risk substances in raw materials, manufacturing processes and other processes to ensure that the residues meet the safety requirements under the intended use conditions, and ensure stability between batches, or carry out substitution studies for high-risk substances. Secondly, sufficient risk assessment should be carried out on leachable substances that may be introduced into the final product in each link, such as monomer, solvent, catalyst, crosslinking agent, etc., as well as some by-products that may appear in the preparation of raw materials, such as naphthalene, which may appear in the preparation of divinylbenzene, etc.

71. Q: In the clearance test of high-throughput haemodialyzer products, whether β_2 microglobulin clearance test conditions can be set to only one blood flow rate, not cover all the blood flow rate range?

A: The clearance rate is the main functional parameter of the hemodialyzer and a key indicator for evaluating the quality of the dialyzer. The clearance rates of urea, creatinine, phosphate, and vitamin B_{12} are commonly used as indicators to evaluate the filtration performance of dialyzers. For high-flux hemodialyzers, β_2 microglobulin clearance performance tests or clinical evaluation data should also be provided. According to YY0053 *Hemodialysis and relevant therapies—Haemodialysers, haemodiafilters, haemofilters and haemoconcentrators*, in the high-flux hemodialyzer, a single blood flow rate can be selected to evaluate the clearance rate of β_2 microglobulin under the blood flow rate commonly used in clinical practice.

72. Q: How to understand the exclusion of infusion products from *Catalogue of Medical Devices Exempted from Clinical Evaluation*?

A: *Catalogue of Medical Devices Exempted from Clinical Evaluation* stipulates that exemptions do not include new materials, new mechanisms of action or new functions including conditions that have not been used in the same type of infusion devices on the market in China.

(1) New materials, such as TOTM plasticizer for PVC raw material of infusion set pipeline, have been used in similar products on the market. Infusion sets made of TOTM plasticizer PVC raw materials do not belong to the category of new materials and can be exempted from clinical evaluation of the product.

(2) New mechanism of action, such as infusion device using floating or membrane type liquid stop components, and the same components have been used in similar products on the market. When applying for registration, the mechanism of action does not belong to the category of new mechanism of action, which can be exempted from clinical evaluation of the product.

(3) In terms of new functions, for example, infusion needle has the function of preventing puncture, and the same function has been used in similar products on the market, which does not belong to the category of new functions when applying for registration, and can be exempted from clinical evaluation of this product.

73. Q: How to evaluate the risk of medical devices containing nanomaterials?

A: Medical devices containing nanomaterials should comply with the risk factors specified in GB/T 16886.1 *Biological evaluation of medical devices—Part 1: Evaluation and testing within a risk management process*, YY/T 0316 *Medical devices—Application of risk management to medical devices* and *Guidance for Technical Review and Registration of Medical Device Products Benefit-Risk Assessment*, mainly including the possibility of release of nanomaterials from the devices, and dose, route, location and duration of exposure. The possibility of release of nanomaterials from medical devices plays the most important factor in risk assessment. Risk assessment should be conducted in a phased, step-by-step manner, considering exposure (nanomaterial release) assessment, distribution and persistence of nanomaterial and environmental transformation, hazard identification, and ultimately a comprehensive assessment of the risk based on whether the scope of application of the product provides sufficient benefits to patients.

74. Q: How to consider the safety of medical devices containing nanomaterials?

A: Due to difference in specific surface area and other factors, nanomaterials exhibit unique physical and chemical properties. Therefore, organisms exposed to nanomaterials may exhibit different biological reactions from bulk materials. The applicant should design a series of tests to confirm the applicability of the test system according to the structural characteristics of the medical device, the intended use, the way of contact with the human body, and the types and forms of the nanomaterials contained in the medical device, so as to establish a biological evaluation plan suitable for the characteristics of the declared product. The biological evaluation system of GB/T 16886 *Biological evaluation of medical devices* series of standards are generally applicable to nanomaterials, but the test method, sample preparation, cell line/animal line selection, observation endpoint and result analysis of a specific medical device using nanomaterials may be different from bulk materials.

75. Q: What are the product performance indicators of high-pressure contrast injector and accessory products?

A: Product performance include but are not limited to the following: appearance, cases and protective cap should not come off naturally and can be easily removed, isolation with the outside world (if applicable), ruhr cone joint meet the requirements of series of standards GB/T 1962 *Conical fittings with a 6% (Luer) taper for syringes, needles and certain other medical equipment*, particle pollution, imaging syringe (lubricant, transparency, the dial with logo, taper joint, seal), the piercing type drug absorption cork puncture and inlet device meet the requirements of YY 0804 *Transfer sets for pharmaceutical preparations—Requirements and test methods*, tubular drug absorption is suitable for the syringe and the wall thickness is not less than 0.5mm, connecting pipe (size, connected firmly, and sex, one-way valve), extractable metal content, pH, readily oxidized, ethylene oxide residues (if applicable), sterility, bacterial endotoxins. The suitability study data of the application product and the high-pressure contrast injection equipment should be submitted.

76. Q: Do biological evaluation of subchronic toxicity, genotoxicity, and implantation evaluation have to be required for registration of single-use epidural catheterization?

A: According to GB/T 16886.1 *Biological evaluation of medical devices—Part 1: Evaluation and testing within a risk management process*, sub-chronic toxicity, genotoxicity and implantation evaluation are not required for epidural catheter products that have been in contact with the human body for less than 30 days. Subchronic toxicity, genotoxicity, and implantation evaluations are required for products used for advanced cancer epidural analgesia, such as epidural catheters for advanced cancer analgesia, that have been in continuous contact with humans for more than 30 days .

77. Q: How to verify the matching performance of disposable endoscope injection needle and endoscope?

A: The administrative counterpart should clarify the size of the endoscopic forceps channel recommended for use with each type of endoscopic injection needle. Provide research data on fit performance, including when simulating clinical use about using the product with endoscopic needle endoscope (or endoscopy simulation pliers, which should be proved compliant with clinical practice) can free access, no obvious resistance, card plug, distortions, operation is flexible and various components conform to the requirements of the use, the needle and armhole are normal smoothly for many times, and there is no bad phenomena such as fracture and detachment at the connecting part.

78. Q: What are the minimum contents included in the performance study of the citric acid disinfectant used for sterilizing the internal pipelines of the hemodialysis machine?

A: The main component of the citric acid disinfectant used for heating and sterilizing the internal pipelines of the hemodialysis machine is citric acid, and can generally also contain lactic acid and malic acid. The performance research of this type of product at least includes: appearance, pH, loading, main active ingredients of the product (such as citric acid), validity period, corrosiveness to metals, and indicators of sterilization of microorganisms, etc. If the main active ingredient of the product contains special substances, or other functions that are not similar to the listed products, the composition, content and performance of the corresponding substances should be specified.

79. Q: What are the requirements for raw materials for Vaseline gauze?

A: Vaseline gauze is generally used for wound protection and packing of burns, scalds, the donor area and skin graft area of skin transplantation, and exuding wounds that require drainage. YY/T 1293.1 *Contacting wound dressing—Part 1: Paraffin Gauze* specifies the performance requirements for this type of product. Vaseline should meet the requirements of the Pharmacopoeia of the People's Republic of China. For imported products, refer to the requirements of the US Pharmacopoeia or the European Pharmacopoeia. For absorbent cotton gauze or absorbent cotton viscose blended gauze, it is recommended to refer to YY0331 *Performance requirements and test methods for absorbent cotton gauze and absorbent cotton and viscose gauze.*

80. Q: What should be considered about biological evaluation of blood purification products for patients with renal failure?

A: Referring to the series of standards of GB/T 16886 *Biological evaluation of medical devices*, the overall biological evaluation should consider the following aspects:

(1) Materials used for manufacture.

(2) Anticipated additives, process contaminants and residues.

(3) Leachable substances.

(4) Degradation products (if applicable).

(5) Other components and their interactions in the final product.

(6) The performance and characteristics of the final product.

(7) Physical properties of the final product, including but not limited to: porosity, particle size, properties and surface morphology.

(8) According to the intended clinical use of the blood purification product, the biological evaluation of the product should take into account the cumulative action time, and be carried out in accordance with the requirements for permanent contact between externally connected devices and circulating blood. It is also recommended that the relevant endpoints be considered in the risk assessment if the product uses a completely new material, or may contain substances that are carcinogenic, mutagenic and reproductively toxic.

Chapter 3

Common technical issues of in vitro diagnostic reagents

81. Q: What is the test system of IVD reagents? If the IVD reagents do not contain all the components of the test system during the registration process, is it necessary to specify the test system of the products?

A: The test system of IVD reagent is composed of the sample processing products, detection reagents, calibrators, controls, detection equipment, etc., which can complete all steps from sample processing to final result report. The whole test system has been fully evaluated for safety and effectiveness and be approved.

During the registration process of IVD reagent, it may not include other products needed to complete the test, in which case the supporting products should be specified in the instructions to ensure that the test process is carried out according to the test system composed of all the conformed supporting products. For example, for nucleic acid detection reagents that do not include extraction reagents, the extraction reagents claimed in the instructions should be used in the process of performance evaluation and clinical evaluation.

Similarly, if comparison reagent is involved in the application data, it is necessary to be operated according to the approved test system of it. If the extraction reagent which is not claimed in the instruction is used to extract nucleic acid and do the following tests, the results have not been fully verified and confirmed, and cannot be used as the comparison of the candidate reagent.

82. Q: For IVD reagents based on next-generation sequencing, do the pre-library preparation reagents have to be included in the composition of the kit for registration?

A: The pre-library preparation reagents generally include the components related to the preparation of the pre library such as end repair, connector connection and amplification, which are used to complete the general processing of the gene sequencing library. After that, other components in the kit need to be used for the specific identification or enrichment of the library. The preparation step of the pre library is a key step in the detection based on the next-generation sequencing and the quality of the pre library preparation reagents affects the accuracy of the detection results directly. Therefore, the administrative counterparts should include the pre library preparation reagents in the composition of the kit for registration, in order to control the stability of the product.

It is worth noting, all the pre-library preparation reagents defined in the classification catalog are class Ⅲ medical device. Therefore, the pre-library preparation reagents cannot be separated for filing.

83. Q: What circumstances require a cybersecurity test report during the IVD equipment registration?

A: According to the *Guidance for premarket review of medical devices cybersecurity*, administrative counterparts need specify the requirements of data interface and user access control in the product technical requirements. If the product is approved before the release of this guidance, without including the above requirements, it is suggested to submit an application for change registration to supplement the relevant indicators. When applying for other changes, if the content of cybersecurity is involved, it is necessary for the administrative counterparts to specify the indicators of cybersecurity in the product technical requirements. In the above two cases, the test report of supplementary items and the cybersecurity description document should be submitted as the supporting data.

84. Q: What documents need to be submitted for the change registration of the packing specifications of IVD reagents?

A: If the packing specifications of IVD reagents are changed, the differences between before and after change of the packing specifications should be described in detail. According to the specific differences, all relevant potential risks should be identified, and these risk factors should be analyzed and verified. For example, ① if there are differences in the reaction form (such as drugs detection products) and reaction film size (such as PCR amplification and hybridization products) between before and after change, the analysis and evaluation data of the changed packing specification should be submitted; ② if the filling volume or container is changed significantly, resulting in increased risks such as evaporation and loss, the changes of the shelf life, in-use stability and calibration frequency should be considered.

85. Q: What contents should be included in " (*II*) *Overview*: *describe the change in detail, the specific reason and purpose of the change*" in the change registration application of IVD reagents?

A: when applying for change registration, the reason and purpose of the change are supposed to be described in detail, and the root cause of the change should be explained. For the products whose performance claims to be improved, how to improve the performance through optimization should be described in detail. For the reason of instruction change of the imported product, when it is described as "updating according to the original instruction" , the reason for the change of the original instruction should also be explained. It is recommended to describe the change in detail, list all design changes of the product, and state that the rest have not changed.

86. Q: How can procalcitonin detection reagents be exempted from clinical trials?

A: Procalcitonin detection reagents are used for the quantitative determination of procalcitonin in human serum or plasma samples in vitro. Procalcitonin detection reagents have been included in the *Catalogue of IVD Reagents Exempted from Clinical Trials*. The intended use of procalcitonin detection reagents in the catalogue is to detect the content of procalcitonin (PCT) in human samples, which is mainly used for auxiliary diagnosis of bacterial infectious diseases in clinical practice. Administrative counterparts who applying for procalcitonin detection reagents for auxiliary diagnosis of bacterial infectious diseases, including auxiliary diagnosis of bacterial infections of different degrees, can apply according to the clinical-free evaluation path. If administrative counterparts apply for other intended uses of procalcitonin detection reagents, which is not within the scope of the *Catalogue of IVD Reagents Exempted from Clinical Trials*, clinical trials are needed to validate the intended uses.

87. Q: For IVD reagents based on ELISA, does the reaction mode have to be changed from "two-step method" to "one-step method" by changing the registration?

A: The ELISA method includes one-step method and two-step method according to the reaction mode. The one-step method is to add the sample and the enzyme-labeled antibody to the reaction well for reaction in the same time, while the two-step method is to add the sample to the reaction well first, and then add the enzyme-labeled antibody after the first reaction completed. The experimental steps of the two methods are different. The former shortens the reaction time, but might degrade product performance. Therefore, changing the two-step method to one-step method by changing the registration is not recommended.

88. Q: What need to do if the instruction of a medical device changes?

A: According to Article 16 of *Regulations on the Administration of Instruction and Label of Medical Devices*, when an approved medical device is changed, the applicant should amend the instruction and label on his own according to the approved change document. If the changed contents of instruction is not specified in the registration certificate and its attachments, which is not within the scope of change registration, it should be notified in writing to the approval department for medical device registration, and submit relevant documents including comparison statements on the change of the instruction.

89. Q: Can the interference test results of qualitative detection reagents only be expressed as negative or positive?

A: The interference test generally adopts the method of pairing comparison, and compares the difference of the test results of the samples containing high concentrations of interfering substances and the samples without or containing normal concentrations of interfering substances (controls). For qualitative detection reagents whose results have no quantitative data, the interference test results can only be expressed as negative or positive, but it should be noted that the research samples should contain weak positive levels. For qualitative detection reagents based on quantitative data (such as OD value, Ct value, or counting results) for threshold judgment, it is recommended to perform differential analysis on quantitative data, rather than just using negative or positive to express the results of the interference test.

90. Q: Which reagents have been adjusted management category in the Announcement on the Adjustment of Part of the *6840 IVD Reagents Classification Sub-Catalogue* (*Edition 2013*)?

A: In October 2020, the NMPA issued the Announcement on the Adjustment of Part of the *6840 IVD Reagents Classification*

Sub-Catalog (*Edition 2013*) (*No.112 of 2020*), which adjusted the management category of some tumor marker related reagents used for treatment monitoring to class II, while the tumor marker related reagents used for auxiliary diagnosis in the *6840 IVD Reagents Classification Sub-Catalog* (*Edition 2013*) have not been adjusted and continue to be managed according to class III.

91. Q: How to standardize the format of the instruction for use of the 2019-nCoV Antigen Test Kit?

A: Except to meet the requirements of the *Guideline for the In-vitro diagnostic reagents instructions compilation*, the instruction for use of the 2019-nCoV Antigen Test Kit also need to combine the enclosure of the *Guideline for the registration of 2019-nCoV Antigen Test Kit*, which is the template of 2019-nCoV Antigen Test Kit (xxxx method) instruction, with the performance of itself, to standardize the format. For example, the intended use, sampling steps, sampling considerations, test method considerations, limitations, etc. For the content of italics, bold, underline in the template, the instruction for use of the 2019-nCoV Antigen Test Kit should also be consistent with it.

92. Q: In the research of clinical items performance for polymerase-chain-reaction (PCR) test equipment, Do the reagents for evaluation have to be approved?

A: The purpose of the research of clinical items performance for PCR test equipment is to evaluate the analytical performance of the whole detection system of equipment and reagents on representative clinical items. The matching reagents used for evaluation should be mature and reliable. Generally, the reagents for evaluation must be marketed. Standard PCR test equipment is open platform, which can support a variety of marketed reagents. For special PCR test equipment, if there are no marketed reagents, it is allowed to use unapproved but finalized reagents for research.

93. Q: What are the requirements for storage conditions for the stability research of IVD reagents?

A: The stability of IVD reagents is the ability to maintain its performance characteristics within the limits specified by the manufacturer.

When conducting the stability research of reagents, full consideration should be given to variables that may affect the properties or effectiveness of reagents. Changes in environmental factors should be taken into account, including the worst case. During the research, reagents should be stored under the conditions specified by the manufacturer, which need to be set according to the capabilities of the equipment used for testing or the expected storage conditions of reagents, and which should adequately verify the stability of reagents under the most unfavorable conditions. The research results should be able to demonstrate that declared reagents can meet the stability requirements under the claimed storage conditions and time. It is recommended that the administrative counterpart should specify the specific range of storage conditions in the research documents and stability claims (e.g., stored at 2-8°C), rather than using indefinite words such as refrigerated, frozen or room temperature to describe storage temperatures.

94. Q: Is it necessary that stability indicators should be included in performance indicators in the technical requirements of IVD reagents?

A: According to Article 4 "Requirements for performance indicators" of the *Guidance for Product Technical Requirements of Medical Device*, the shelf-life of medical devices belongs to research and evaluation contents which are not recommended to be specified in performance indicators in the technical requirements. This suggestion also applies to the product technical requirements of IVD reagents. Stability may not be included in performance indicators in the product technical requirements of IVD reagents.

95. Q: How to choose a comparator method for bacterial drug resistance gene detection reagent in clinical trials?

A: Bacterial drug resistance gene detection reagents are the kind of reagents, which detect the specific resistance genes of target bacteria to determine its resistance to the drug. In clinical trial for this kind of reagents, the applicant should first choose the results of clinical drug resistance phenotype as a clinical reference standard as the comparator method. By comparing with the clinical drug resistance test result, the sensitivity and specificity of gene detection reagent to drug resistant bacteria are obtained. The performance of the reagents in detecting relevant genes in clinical samples can be confirmed by comparison with gene sequencing or similar products approved by NMPA.

For the reagents whose drug resistance gene site are widely

recognized in clinical application, and whose similar products have been approved for many years, can mainly compare with the similar products approved. Some samples can be further confirmed by comparison with drug resistance phenotypes for the clinical trial. The applicant should refer to the guidances if there are applicable ones.

96. Q: Can the cut off or reference intervals be adjusted in clinical trial of IVD reagents?

A: The establishment and verification for the cut off or reference interval of IVD reagents is generally completed before the clinical trial, and the clinical trial results are interpreted according to the fully validated cut off or reference interval. If the cut off or reference interval of the IVD reagent is unreasonable and needs to be adjusted according to the clinical reference standard in the clinical trial, the adjusted data would be used as the cut off or reference interval study data, rather than the clinical research data to confirm the clinical performance of the product. The clinical subjects should be renewed for clinical trial after adjustment.

97. Q: Can the retest results be included in the final consistency statistics for samples with inconsistent test results of the investigational reagents and comparator reagents during the clinical trials of IVD reagents?

A: During the clinical trials of IVD reagents, in order to control the test bias, the test results which be used for the statistical analysis of the consistency of the investigational reagents and comparator, should be the results before unblinding. For inconsistent samples, if the re-test is carried out according to the clinical trial protocol, the re-test results if included in the statistical analysis will introduce bias. Therefore, it is not recommended to include the re-test results in the overall statistical analysis. However, combination the re-test results with the test results of the third-party review reagents and the clinical diagnosis information of the corresponding subjects of the samples, can be used for further analysis of the reasons for the inconsistency of the test results.

98. Q: What are the concerns of product instructions in clinical trials of IVD reagents?

A: During the design and implementation of clinical trials of IVD reagents, special attention should be paid to the consistency of operational details in the clinical trial process with the relevant product instructions, including instructions for investigational reagents, comparator reagents, and review reagents.

Whether it is an investigational reagents reagent, a comparator reagent, or a review reagent, the contents of the instructions that should be concerned to in clinical trials include intended use, applicable sample types, anticoagulants used in samples, sample preservation and processing requirements, and supporting reagents for sample processing (such as nucleic acid extraction reagents) and other supporting reagents, applicable instruments, test methods, results interpretation standards, limitations, etc. In the process of clinical trial design, detailed standard operating procedures should be formulated in accordance with the relevant instructions to ensure that the detection of investigational reagents, comparator reagents, and review reagents in the clinical trial is strictly in accordance with the requirements of the instructions, and the clinical trial testing process and results should be able to support the claimed content of investigational reagent instructions.

99. Q: What are the concerns when submitting ethical documents and clinical trial protocols for registration application of IVD reagents?

A: The applicant should submit the clinical trial protocol implemented and the review documents of the ethics committees approved carrying out the clinical trial when submitting the clinical trial documents.

Due to the clinical trial protocol revision, there may be several version numbers. The following principles should be noted when submitting application documents:

If the clinical trial protocol is revised before the clinical trial, the protocol for the final implementation in the clinical trial and the approval documents of the ethics committee for this version number protocol should be submitted.

If the clinical trial has already started and the protocol revision occurs during the trial, the final version of the clinical trial protocol and informed consent form, and the approval documents of the ethics committee for previous revisions have to be submitted. The clinical trial protocol with the final version should list the previous revisions in detail. If not listed, the clinical trial protocols of the previous revisions have to be submitted. The applicant should explain the reasons for the revisions of the protocol and the impact on the clinical trials that have been conducted clearly.

It should be noted that the scientificity, rationality, feasibility and compliance of the protocol should be fully studied before the clinical trial, and the protocol should be formulated and strictly implemented. During the clinical trial, the protocol should not be arbitrarily changed for non-essential reasons.

100. Q: What are the requirements for anticoagulants used in samples in IVD clinical trials?

A: When the different anticoagulants are used in test samples of IVD reagents, the anticoagulants should be studied in the pre-clinical research to verify the applicability of them and their impact on the detection. In general, if the pre-clinical study indicates that the available anticoagulants in the instructions don't have the differential impact on sample detection, there is no need to enroll samples using different anticoagulants in the clinical trial, and all applicable anticoagulants can be used in clinical trial samples. In some special cases, if different anticoagulants have a significant impact on the test results, resulting in different reference values for the determination of clinical test results, samples collection and research should be validated separately in clinical trials. The sample types and the anticoagulants used in the samples should be clearly stated in the clinical trial protocol and report.

101. Q: What should be paid attention to the samples in clinical trials of IVD reagents?

A: Sample is a very critical element in clinical trials of IVD reagents. In clinical trials, the sponsor should concern on sample collection, storage conditions, storage time, processing methods, etc. The whole-process management of samples have to meet the requirements of the instructions for investigational reagents and comparator reagents. For example, in the clinical trial of nucleic acid detection reagents, should pay attention to :

(1) The original clinical samples should be used for clinical trials, and the extracted DNA or RNA nucleic acid should not be regarded as the original sample.

(2) Nucleic acid extraction/purification reagents and sample preservation solution (if applicable) used in clinical trials have to meet the requirements of the instructions for investigational reagents and comparator reagents.

(3) If the product instructions require the purity and concentration of the extracted nucleic acid, they should meet the relevant requirements of the respective product instructions.

(4) Sample storage conditions and storage time should meet the requirements.

(5) Operations such as sample collection tube, preservation solution, and inactivation should meet the requirements of the instructions, too.

102. Q: What factors should be considered in the coverage of gene mutation sites during the development of non-original companion diagnostic reagents for anti-tumor drugs?

A: For non-original companion diagnostic gene mutation detection reagents for anti-tumor drugs, the selection of genes and the coverage of the gene sites in product design should be fully considered during product development. If the gene is known to have multiple mutation sites for the same companion diagnostic use (such as the same companion drug), the subsequent product design should fully consider the coverage of the mutation sites in combination with the product risk-benefit analysis. The applicant could not narrow the detection range of the gene sites just for evaluating the product easily. For example, when *KRAS* gene mutation is used for tumor companion diagnosis, which is a negative companion diagnostic gene test and is related to adverse drug reactions. Insufficient coverage of the mutation sites may increase the risk of patients, so the applicant should fully refer to the original companion diagnostic reagents or the gene coverage in drug clinical trials.

103. Q: What are the concerns when using overseas clinical trial data of IVD reagents for registration?

A: The applicant should submit the ethical opinion, clinical trial protocol and clinical trial report of the overseas clinical trial institution, when using overseas clinical trial data as clinical evidence for registration application in our country. The form, content and signature of ethical documents, clinical trial protocols and reports should meet the relevant requirements of clinical trial quality management in the country (region) where the overseas clinical trial is located. In addition, the applicant should also submit a difference analysis report on the relevant factors of domestic and foreign clinical trials. In this report, the applicant should describe detailed the differences between the relevant factors in the overseas clinical trials of the investigational reagent and those in China and measures for the differences. When necessary, the relevant laws, regulations, norms or standards of the country (region) where the overseas clinical trial is located should also be submitted.

The applicant should provide complete overseas clinical trial data without screening, and the overseas clinical trial report should include the analysis and conclusion of the complete clinical trial data.

104. Q: How should the inclusion and exclusion criteria for subjects in the clinical trial design of in IVD reagents be formulated?

A: In IVD clinical trials, reasonable subject inclusion and exclusion criteria should be set according to the applicable population and indications for the intended use of the product. It should be noted that clinical trial subjects should be from the applicable population (target population) and indications claimed for the intended use of the product, such as those with certain symptoms, signs, physiology, pathological conditions or certain epidemiological backgrounds. Enrollment of non-target populations may introduce subject selection bias, resulting in clinical trial results that cannot reflect the real situation of the product.

For example, for IVD reagents used for auxiliary diagnosis of certain diseases, a large number of asymptomatic healthy subjects should not be randomly enrolled in clinical trials. A large number of the preoperative screening of patients without related symptoms and signs should not be enrolled in clinical trials of hepatitis B, hepatitis C, AIDS, syphilis and other related detection reagents. Because the above inclusion criteria may cause the clinical specific evaluation of the product to deviate from the true performance of the product.

105. Q: What key points should be concerned when the companion diagnostic reagent is used as the clinical evidence of the companion diagnostic through the bridging test pathway?

A: The bridging test is to use the investigational reagents to test the remaining samples of patients enrolled during the completed key drug clinical trials, and then evaluate the therapeutic effect of the subjects determined by the investigational reagents.

When the companion diagnostic reagent is used as the clinical evidence of the companion diagnostic through the bridging test pathway, attention should be paid to:

（1）The pivotal drug clinical trial supporting the domestic marketing of the drug should be confirmed first, and the bridging trial should include the remaining samples of all enrolled cases in the pivotal clinical trial. Insufficient amount, lack of informed consent, etc., part of it is allowed to drop out, but the amount of shedding should not affect the overall evaluation.

（2）If the drug clinical trial is an international multi-center clinical trial, the bridging trial should include not only the remaining samples of domestic cases, but also the remaining samples of all overseas cases.

（3）If the drug clinical trial is an enrichment trial design, the enrolled cases may only be those with positive marker detection result, or the negative cases in the drug clinical trial are insufficient, the bridging test should exclude the enrolled cases of the drug clinical trial. In addition to the remaining samples, some case samples from non-drug clinical trials need to be included to evaluate the clinical performance of the test in vitro diagnostic reagents and the original companion diagnostic reagents or CTA. The entry and excretion criteria for this part of the supplementary cases should be strictly set, and should be the applicable population for the test in vitro diagnostic reagents. For this part of the additionally enrolled negative samples, the test in vitro diagnostic reagents and the original research companion diagnostic reagents or CTA need to be tested simultaneously.

106. Q: What issues should be paid attention to when submitting IVDs clinical trial database?

A: In accordance with the requirements of the *Announcement on the Announcement of In Vitro Diagnostic Reagent Registration Application Materials Requirements and Approval Document Format* (*No. 122 of 2021*) , the clinical trial database should be submitted for all IVD reagents that undergo clinical evaluation through the clinical trial from January 1st, 2022. Applicants should submit the clinical trial database correctly in accordance with the requirements of the *Guidelines for Submission of Registration Review of Clinical Trial Data of In Vitro Diagnostic Reagents.* The clinical trial database should include the original database, analysis database, descriptive documents, program code (if has) .

The original database refers to the information of all cases and samples enrolled in the clinical trial according to the requirements of the protocol, including the cases that were excluded during the trial, and the reasons for the exclusion should be noted. the applicant should provide the original data sets of each institution and the aggregated original data sets.

Analysis database refers to a database formed by using original data sets for statistical analysis, which is used to generate statistical results in clinical trial reports, and should include corresponding case and sample information for statistical analysis. Analysis database usually composed of multiple different data sets, which formation should correspond to the statistical results in the clinical trial report.

The descriptive documents should at least include data description documents and statistical analysis documents. Depending on the statistical analysis tool used, the statistical analysis process should be articulated in the statistical analysis documentation to facilitate data re-examination during the review process. For data management based on the EDC system, an annotated case report form must also be submitted.

If program code is used in database management or statistical analysis, the program code should be provided, including the code used for generating the analysis database from the original database, and the code for generating statistical results from the analysis database, etc. It should be noted that, while providing the program code, the applicant should also explain the use method, system and software environment of the program code file in the statistical analysis document, including whether and how to modify the program code when using the code file. And the program code files and data set file names used to generate each statistical result chart are listed one by one in tabular form.

The original database and analysis database can be submitted in excel form, but it should be noted that the applicant should not only submit an excel form consistent with the data summary table in the clinical application materials, but also submit the analysis database and descriptive documents according to the above requirements.

Chapter 4

Other general technological issues

107. Q: For a product which has undergone clinical evaluation through clinical evaluation of the predicate device or through clinical trial, if it has been included into the *Catalogue of Medical Devices Exempted from Clinical Trials*, can the applicant change the clinical evaluation path when supplementing the data?

A: For a medical device under review which has undergone clinical evaluation through clinical evaluation of the predicate device or through clinical trial, if the declared product is listed in the officially released *Catalogue of Medical Devices Exempted from Clinical Trials*. The applicant can, according to its needs, prove the safety and effectiveness of the product from the aspects of basic principle, structure, performance, safety, scope of application, etc., in accordance with the *Technical Guidance for Comparison Description of products in the Catalogue of Medical Devices Exempted from Clinical evaluation*. In this case, considering that the clinical evaluation data in the supplementary data have been changed significantly compared with the initial submission, the applicant can make full use of the post-supplementation consultation and pre-review and other communications to fully communicate with the reviewers.

108. Q: Can the clinical evaluation of liquid products for in vitro assisted reproduction be conducted through clinical evaluation of the predicate device?

A: Some liquid products for in vitro assisted reproduction have been included into the *Catalogue of Medical Devices Exempted from Clinical Trials*, and it's recommended to select appropriate clinical evaluation path for those not included into the catalogue, including clinical trial and clinical evaluation of the predicate device. If an enterprise intends to apply for registration through clinical evaluation of the predicate device, the following conditions can be considered for comprehensive evaluation:

(1) Considering the diversity of components of liquid products for in vitro assisted reproduction, if the components of the selected single predicate device cannot cover all components of the proposed product during the comparison of components, it can be considered to add the predicate device to cover the components of the proposed product that cannot be covered by a single predicate device.

(2) For the concentration difference of common basic components such as normal saline component, energy substrate, acid-base buffer system, amino acid, human serum albumin, and antibiotics, if the concentration of each component of the predicate device cannot be obtained, and the influence of the concentration difference of the above components on safety and effectiveness can be reflected through comparison of performance indicators, such as pH value, osmotic pressure, impurity limit, use performance indicator, and mouse embryo test, concentration comparison information may not be provided. For specific functional components related to the intended use, concentration comparison information should be provided and the impact of difference on safety and effectiveness should be evaluated.

(3) During clinical evaluation of the predicate device, it should be noted in adopting clinical literature data and clinical experience data that the evaluation indicators should reflect the clinical use of the product and the clinical outcomes related to the product, such as fertilization rate, cleavage rate, blastocyst rate, implantation rate, pregnancy rate and other applicable indicators.

109. Q: For surgical navigation system used to guided percutaneous needle or tracking and navigation surgical instrument by optical tracking and/or electromagnetic tracking technology, is it necessary to provide clinical evaluation data based on clinical trials?

A: Whether clinical trials should be conducted for such products can be comprehensively determined based on the clinical function, scope of application, adequacy of existing non-clinical verification and the situation of the product approved for marketing in China. For example, it can be considered to conduct the clinical evaluation of the following two types of products through comparison with the predicate device.

First, preoperative image-guided percutaneous needle for insertion into the chest and abdomen (including biopsy needle and ablation needle), which generally includes needle-holding robotic arm, which can insert the needle through the needle placement path confirmed by the doctor.

Second, tracking and navigation surgical instrument, which is used to guide physicians to perform surgical operations according to patients' preoperative images, does not include robotic arm, and generally has the functions of preoperative approach planning of surgical instrument and multi-modal image registration/fusion. It's recommended to consider providing data on bench test, animal test and clinical literature of similar products to demonstrate the safety and effectiveness of the product on the basis of full comparison and analysis of the similarities and differences between the proposed product and the predicate device in clinical functions, performance parameters, etc. When necessary, cadaver test data in line with relevant management requirements can also be considered.

110. Q: According to the guidelines, when conducting clinical evaluation through clinical trial, in addition to providing overseas clinical trial data, clinical trial still needs to be conducted in China. Does the applicant need to conduct clinical trial?

A: As specified in Clause 5 of *Technical Guidelines for Accepting Overseas Clinical Trials of Medical Devices*, "If the technical review guidelines for a particular medical device contain relevant clinical trial requirements, such requirements should be considered for the overseas clinical trial of the medical device. In case of any inconsistency, sufficient and reasonable grounds and basis should be provided" Therefore, if the applicant has submitted clinical trial data conforming to ethical, legal and scientific principles in accordance with the *Technical Guidelines for Accepting Overseas Clinical Trials of Medical Devices*, and has fully considered differences in technical review requirements, subject populations and clinical trial conditions, additional clinical trials may not be conducted in China.

111. Q: How to choose the clinical evaluation path when applying for registration of hip prosthesis products? What issues should be paid attention to when choosing clinical evaluation of the predicate device?

A: When applying for registration of hip prosthesis products, appropriate clinical evaluation path can be selected based on the specific scope of application and technical characteristics of the proposed product. Generally speaking, if there is any predicate device with the same scope of application and similar technical characteristics (such as mechanism of action, materials, design, and product performance) which has been marketed in China, the registration applicant can consider clinical evaluation of the predicate device. In case of clinical evaluation of the predicate device for hip prosthesis, the applicable part of *Technical Guidelines for Clinical Evaluation of Medical Devices* should be complied with. It is recommended to pay attention to the following items:

(1) Selection of the predicate device. Products that have been marketed in China with the same scope of application and the same or similar technical characteristics as the proposed product should be selected as far as possible as predicate devices. If the selected predicate device is significantly different from the proposed product, more scientific evidence should be provided to demonstrate that the difference does not adversely affect the safety and effectiveness of the product. The applicant is encouraged to conduct comprehensive research on marketed similar products when choosing the predicate device.

(2) Comparison between the proposed product and the predicate device.It is necessary to make clear the same scope of application and technical characteristics of the proposed product and the predicate device, and elaborate on the similarities and differences between the two products.

(3) Provision of clinical data on the predicate device.The applicant should make clear the relevance of clinical data to the predicate device. It is suggested that the applicant extract key elements from clinical literature for subsequent data analysis.

(4) Provision of scientific evidence for differences. Based on the specific differences between the proposed product and the predicate device, appropriate scientific evidence should be submitted, such as non-clinical study data and/or clinical data on the proposed product, including non-clinical study data and/or clinical data that can represent the proposed product.

112. Q: Since the clinical trial protocol has been revised many times during the trial process, is it necessary to submit all previous trial protocols, opinions of the ethics committee and informed consent forms when submitting product registration?

A: The final version of the clinical trial protocol and informed consent form as well as opinions of ethics committee on all previous changes should be submitted. All previous changes should be listed in detail in the final version of the clinical trial protocol; if not, all previously changed clinical trial protocols should be submitted. The applicant should provide reasons for changing the clinical trial protocol.

113. Q: Is it necessary to use all models and specifications of the proposed product for the clinical trial?

A: It is suggested to analyze the differences among different models of the proposed product based on its scope of application, objective of the clinical trial, evaluation indicators, etc. At the same time, combined with the results of the model and specification of the proposed product, it should be comprehensively evaluated whether the models and specifications used in the clinical trial are representative of all the models and specifications of the proposed product.

114. Q: If the clinical trial protocol of a product includes feasibility trial and confirmatory trial, can the results of feasibility trial and confirmatory clinical trial be combined for statistics after the trial?

A: Feasibility trial can make an initial assessment of product safety and performance to provide information for confirmatory trial design, and is different from confirmatory clinical trial in terms of objective. The statistics of test results should follow the prescribed statistical analysis plan. Therefore, it is not recommended to combine the results of feasibility trial and confirmatory clinical trial for statistics after the trial.

115. Q: In case of failure in applying for renewal of registration within the specified time for a registered product, application for registration of the product should be made according to regulatory requirements. In this case, can the original registered product be selected as the predicate device for clinical evaluation? How should clinical data be provided?

A: In this case, the original registered product can be selected as the predicate device for clinical evaluation. Attention should be mainly paid to whether there is any difference between the proposed product and the original registered product in comparison with the predicate device. If there is no difference between the two products, the clinical data to be provided may include the pre-marketing and post-marketing clinical data of the product, and the clinical experience data including post-marketing adverse events.

116. Q: According to the guidelines for medical device products (excluding *in vitro* diagnostic reagents), if clinical trial still needs to be conducted in China for a product with overseas clinical trial data, and the applicant has submitted clinical trial data conforming to the three basic principles in accordance with the *Technical Guidelines for Accepting Overseas Clinical Trials of Medical Devices* with full consideration given to differences in technical review requirements, subject populations and clinical trial conditions, can the product be exempted from clinical trial in China?

A: Yes. As specified in Clause 5 of *Technical Guidelines for Accepting Overseas Clinical Trials of Medical Devices*, "If the technical review guidelines for a particular medical device contain relevant clinical trial requirements, such requirements should be considered for the overseas clinical trial of the medical device. In case of any inconsistency, sufficient and reasonable grounds and basis should be provided". Therefore, if it can be demonstrated that the conclusions of overseas clinical trial data can be extrapolated to use populations in China and meet the relevant technical requirements for registration in China, the data can be used for clinical evaluation, and there is no need to carry out clinical trial in China.

117. Q: What are the definition and construction principles of target value in the single-arm objective performance criteria clinical trial design of medical devices?

A: For single-arm trial design compared with target value, the target value with clinical significance should be predefined for the primary evaluation indicators, and the effectiveness/safety of the investigational medical device can be evaluated through whether the results of the primary evaluation indicators of single-arm clinical trial is within the predefined scope of the target value. Since there is no control group, clinical trials of single-arm objective performance criteria design cannot validate the superiority, equivalence, or non-inferiority of the investigational medical device, and can only validate that the effectiveness/safety meets the minimum standard recognized in the professional field.

The target value is the minimum standard recognized within a professional field that the effectiveness/safety evaluation indicators should meet, including objective performance criteria (OPC) and performance goal (PG). The target values are generally dichotomous (valid/invalid) indicators and may also be quantitative indicators, including target value and one-sided confidence interval boundary (Generally, it is 97.5% one-sided confidence interval boundary). In making statistical analysis on the clinical trial results, it is necessary to calculate the point estimate values and one-sided confidence interval boundary values of primary evaluation indicators, and to compare these calculated values with the target values.

The construction of target values requires normally a

comprehensive collection of clinical study data with a certain level of quality and a considerable number of cases and a scientific analysis (e.g., meta-analysis). With the improvement of device technology and clinical skills, OPC is subject to change and clinical data needs to be re-analyzed for confirmation.

118. Q: How to consider the design type of clinical trial of computer-aided decision-making products based on deep learning?

A: (1) The single-arm objective performance criteria design can be considered for products that provide auxiliary decision-making advice on triage and referral of a patient after determining whether the patient suffers a target disease, such products do not provide specific lesions, and require professional doctors to review the patient's images again, regardless of negative and positive auxiliary triage results. Such products include computer-aided triage and referral products for patients with various target diseases, such as those for auxiliary triage of diabetic retinopathy, pneumonia and cerebral hemorrhage. The diagnostic accuracy indicators (such as sensitivity and specificity, usually at patient level) of product-assisted triage results can be considered for primary evaluation indicators.

(2) A controlled design is recommended for clinical trials of products for auxiliary detection of lesions of target diseases, such as auxiliary detection products for pulmonary nodule and CT image of fracture. The test group should be detected jointly by physicians and the proposed product, while the control group should be detected by traditional diagnostic methods (such as the clinician's film reading/comprehensive diagnosis). Diagnostic accuracy indicators (such as

sensitivity, specificity, AFROC curve and positive rate; lesion-level sensitivity and patient-level specificity generally considered) can be considered for primary evaluation indicators. The comparison type of clinical trial should reflect benefit-risk acceptability of the product, and it is recommended to consider superiority design. For example, in case of pulmonary nodules larger than 4 mm, the superiority of patient-level specificity and the non-inferiority of lesion-level sensitivity can be considered for CT image-assisted detection software.

119. Q: For ultrasonic soft tissue cutting hemostasis system which can be used for closure of vessels up to 7 mm, is it sufficient to provide *in vitro* burst pressure test and animal test as supporting evidence?

A: According to the *Guidelines for Technical Review of Clinical Evaluation of Predicate Device for Ultrasonic Soft Tissue Cutting Hemostasis System,* due to the relatively high risk and technical difficulty in clinical use of ultrasonic soft tissue cutting hemostasis system which can be used for closure of vessels up to 7 mm, it is suggested to further demonstrate its safety and effectiveness through the clinical data of the proposed product on the basis of *in vitro* burst pressure test and animal test. Clinical trials conducted in China should comply with the relevant requirements of the *Good Clinical Practices for Medical Devices.*

120. Q: Can single-arm objective performance criteria design be selected for clinical trials of intracranial drug-coated balloon dilatation catheter?

A: The point of the single-arm objective performance criteria design is to compare the trial results of the primary evaluation indicators with the available clinical data so as to evaluate the effectiveness/safety of the investigational medical device. As compared with that of parallel control trial, the inherent bias of single group trial is asynchronous control bias, which may cause selection bias, confounding bias, measurement bias and evaluation bias due to asynchrony. Since there is no control group, clinical trials of single-arm objective performance criteria design cannot validate the superiority, equivalence, or non-inferiority of the investigational medical device, and can only validate that the effectiveness/safety meets the minimum standard recognized in the professional field. When the investigational medical device technology is relatively sophisticated and there is a deep understanding of its intended diseases, and it is not feasible to set the control (e.g., there is a significant difference in the risks/benefits of the investigational medical device and existing treatment, it is ethically unfeasible to set a control; and when the existing treatment is not feasible due to the objective conditions), the single-arm objective performance criteria design may be considered. According to the technical development and clinical application status of intracranial drug-coated balloon dilatation catheter, the basic principle of single-arm objective performance criteria design is not met. Therefore, it is suggested to choose RCT design for clinical trial.

121. Q: How to conduct the clinical evaluation of all-suture anchors through comparison with the predicate device?

A: Clinical evaluation of all-suture anchors can be conducted through comparison with the predicate device, and similar products with the same scope of application which have been approved for marketing in China should be selected as predicate devices. The items compared with the predicate device include design principle, structural composition, dimension and specification, operation performance, mechanical performance, etc. The comparison of structure and dimension should include the comparison of structure and dimension in natural state and after retraction of soft anchor, and the similarities and differences in braiding pattern and the thickness of single strand should be made clear. In terms of difference in structure and dimension, it is necessary to explain the reason why a design is selected for the proposed product, and demonstrate that the difference does not adversely affect the safety and effectiveness of the product while considering the subsequent mechanical performance. The comparison of operational performance includes insertion force, whether retraction of soft anchor is easy to cause knots, etc. For non-quantitative operational performance evaluation indicators, if product design verification data show that clinical needs can be met, there is no need to compare with the predicate device. The comparison of mechanical performance includes comparison of dynamic and static fixation performance. The mechanical performance of the proposed product should not be inferior to that of the predicate device. When comparing mechanical performance with the predicate device, attention should be paid to the rationality of test parameters (such as load size and cycle times) and the selection of fixed blocks for mechanical test. If artificial bone is used, it is recommended to determine the composition (such as cortical/cancellous bone composite block), thickness and density of the simulated block according to the bone conditions in clinical use, and the diameter of the test hole should be consistent with the diameter in clinical use. When providing each mechanical test report, it is necessary to clarify the failure mode of each sample. Anchors intended for use at anatomical sites with significantly different biomechanical requirements should be compared separately from anchor types with the same scope of application.

122. Q: Is it necessary to conduct clinical trial for all models and specifications in the same registration unit?

A: In principle, the working principle, scope of application, differences among models and specifications and non-clinical study data of the product should be considered. In addition, it should be confirmed whether the product undergoing clinical trial is typical and able to cover all models and specifications of the proposed product after comprehensive consideration combined with objective and primary evaluation indicators of clinical trial.

123. Q: Since the transcatheter heart valve and the delivery system have undergone clinical trial and marketed in China and only the delivery system has been further improved, without any changes in the transcatheter heart valve, which clinical path is appropriate for application?

A: The applicant should make specific analysis on whether the changes in the delivery system have any impact on product performance and clinical safety, and put emphasis on analyzing whether preclinical study data are sufficient to demonstrate that the differences have no impact on product safety and effectiveness. If the differences are acceptable through analysis and evaluation, and can be supported by non-clinical data and clinical data on overseas similar products with the same improvement, the clinical evaluation can be conducted through clinical evaluation of predicate device.

124. Q: When conducting clinical evaluation through clinical trials, is it necessary and how to submit a clinical evaluation report?

A: If a clinical evaluation report is required, it can be conducted in accordance with the requirements of Chapter Ⅳ of the *Technical Guidelines for Clinical Evaluation Reports on Medical Device Registration and Application*, and the clinical evaluation report can be provided by referring to the format requirements of Chapter Ⅴ .

125. Q: Is it necessary to submit original clinical trial data when submitting overseas clinical trial data for clinical evaluation?

A: Submitting overseas clinical trial data for clinical evaluation must comply with the relevant requirements of the *Technical Guidelines for Receiving Overseas Clinical Trial Data of Medical Devices*, and submit clinical trial data in accordance with the *Guidelines for Registration and Review of Clinical Trial Data Submission Requirements for Medical Devices*, including original databases, analysis databases, explanatory documents, and codes.

126. Q: For products with overseas medical device clinical trial data, if there are also published clinical trial guidelines for corresponding products in China, is it necessary the overseas clinical trial data of the product fully must meet the requirements of the corresponding domestic guidelines?

A: Clinical trials conducted overseas may meet the technical review requirements of the country (region) where the trial is conducted, but may not fully meet the relevant review requirements of China. For example, when designing clinical trials, some countries only require clinical trials to conclude that the device performance reaches a certain observation endpoint; However, when applying for registration in China, it may be required that the performance of the device reach multiple observation endpoints to confirm its effectiveness, and that the safety of the medical device be supported by appropriate evidence. If the State Food and Drug Administration issues technical review guidelines for specific medical devices that contain relevant requirements for their clinical trials, relevant requirements should be considered for overseas clinical trials of the device. If there are inconsistencies, sufficient and reasonable reasons and evidence should be provided.

127. Q: How to choose a clinical evaluation path for medical devices?

A: According to the *Regulations on the Supervision and Administration of Medical Devices*, clinical evaluation of medical devices can be conducted based on product characteristics, clinical risks, existing clinical data, and other situations. The safety and effectiveness of medical devices can be demonstrated through conducting clinical trials, or through analyzing and evaluating clinical literature and clinical data of the same variety of medical devices. The applicant for registration can refer to the *Technical Guidelines for Determining whether to Conduct Clinical Trials of Medical Device*s to determine whether to conduct clinical trials, and select an appropriate clinical evaluation path based on the recent announcement of the *Recommended Clinical Evaluation Paths for Related Products in the Medical Device Classification Catalog* issued by Center For Medical Device Evaluation. NMPA.

128. Q: When conducting clinical evaluation based on clinical data of the same type of medical device, what else can be done if clinical literature of the same type of medical device cannot be retrieved?

A: The collection, analysis, and evaluation of clinical data for the same type of medical device have different roles depending on the design characteristics, key technologies, scope of application, and degree of risk of the declared product, including determining whether the safety and effectiveness of the same type of medical device have been clinically recognized, and whether the risk benefits are within an acceptable range; Fully identify the clinical use risks of the same type of medical device, and provide information for the risk benefit analysis of the declared product; Confirm the residual risks of non clinical studies through clinical data; Provide clinical data for evaluation of test results in some non clinical studies (such as bench tests).

In addition to clinical literature data, clinical experience data and clinical trial data for products of the same variety are also included. Clinical experience data includes completed clinical research data sets, adverse event data sets, and corrective action data sets related to clinical risks. Adverse event data sets can be publicly obtained through complaints and adverse events from regulatory agencies after listing.

In addition, the applicant needs to confirm whether the selected product of the same variety is a product with high clinical attention and recognized safety and effectiveness among similar products, and whether the literature retrieval strategy is appropriate to ensure the comprehensiveness of the retrieval.

129. Q: What factors should be considered for the main evaluation indicators of clinical trials of inferior vena cava filters?

A: The inferior vena cava filter (IVCF) is a device designed to prevent pulmonary embolism (PE) caused by the detachment of emboli from deep venous thrombosis (DVT) in the inferior vena cava system. The position and shape of the inferior vena cava filter during implantation not only affect the effectiveness of filtering emboli, but also are closely related to the risk of use. For example, the displacement and inclination of the filter during implantation, as well as the perforation of the blood vessel wall, not only reduces the filtering effectiveness of the emboli, but also may increase the risk of adverse events. Therefore, the main evaluation indicators generally need to comprehensively consider the above factors, including at least the incidence of pulmonary embolism in patients and the location and shape of filters.

130. Q: When selecting the same variety comparison path for clinical evaluation on personalized abutments or machinable abutments, what type of abutments should be selected as the same type of product?

A: The interface between a personalized abutment or a machinable abutment column and a matching implant is generally a fixed interface. Applicants can choose the corresponding finished abutment for the matching implant as the same type of device for comparison, such as triangular, hexagonal, and plum blossom interface types. For each type, at least one finished abutment is selected for comparison with the same type. Generally, other personalized benches or machinable benches are not selected as products of the same variety, but can be used as comparable devices to compare the machinable range with the declared product.

131. Q: When comparing intracranial aspiration catheters with the same variety, what aspects should be paid attention to in selecting blood vessels and thrombus types in animal experiments?

A: In animal experiments, it is recommended to discuss the representativeness of selected blood vessels in terms of vessel diameter, vessel tortuosity, and vessel wall characteristics. Taking the pig model as an example, we can consider selecting the ascending pharyngeal artery, external carotid artery, common carotid artery, lingual artery, subclavian artery, and other suitable blood vessels. The applicant should explain the reason and basis for the selection of target blood vessels one by one. The selected blood vessels should include at least one blood vessel that supplies intracranial blood to the test animal, and consider the smallest diameter blood vessels and vessels with greater tortuosity that the product is intended to use. Artificial thrombus should consider making different types of thrombus, including soft thrombus, mixed thrombus, and hard thrombus. Mixed thrombus can be used as a representative model of soft thrombus.

132. Q: What are the filling requirements for the remark column in the application form of the special review for innovative medical device?

A: The administrative counterparts should complete the remark column in the application form of the special review for innovative medical device as per below requirements: the administrative counterpart should truthfully fill in the information of experts/

units that related to the relevant interests, including but not limited to physical and chemical index testing, biological performance testing, animal testing, clinical trials, the cooperative researchers, the intellectual property buyers and sellers, etc., and specify the experts that applying for avoidance and state the reasons for their avoidance. If there are experts related to the interests, the name of the specific enterprise and the specific R&D project in which the experts are involved should be specified. The remark column should not be blank, "None" can be filled if there is no relevant content.

133. Q: What are the requirements for the submitted intellectual property certificate documents during the special review for innovative medical devices?

A: According to the relevant provisions listed in the *Special Review Procedures for Innovative Medical Devices*, the intellectual property certification documents submitted in the special review of innovative medical devices should meet below requirements:

（1）If the administrative counterparts have obtained the patent right for invention in China, it is required to provide the copies of the patent authorization certificate, the claim and the specification signed and sealed by theministrative counterpart and the original copy of the patent register issued by the patent competent departments. The application time for special review of innovative medical devices should not exceed 5 years from the date of patent authorization announcement.

（2）If the administrative counterparts obtain the right to use the right of an invention patent in China through the transfer according to law, the original *Record Certificate of Patent License Contract* issued by the competent patent authority should also be provided except for the copies of the patent authorization certificate, the claim, the specification and the patent register held by the patentee.The application time for special review of innovative medical device should not exceed 5 years from the date of patent authorization announcement.

(3) If the invention patent application has been disclosed by *the Patent Administration Department of the State Council* and has not been authorized, the copies of the documents proving that the invention patent has been disclosed (such as the notice of publication of invention patent application, the notice of publication and entry into the substantive review stage of invention patent application, the notice of entry into the substantive review stage of invention patent application, etc.) and the copies of the published version of the claims and the specification signed and sealed by the administrative counterparts should be provided. The patent search and consulting center of *the State Intellectual Property Office* should issue a search report, which indicates that the core technical scheme of the product has novelty and creativity. During the review of an application for a patent for invention, if the claims and the specification are modified at the request of the patent review department, the modified text should be submitted; If the patentee is changed, the supporting documents issued by the competent patent department, such as the copy of the notification of qualified procedures, should be submitted.

134. Q: What are the requirements for signatures and seals when applying for the special review of innovative medical devices for imported products?

A: If there is no special description for the application documents for special review of the imported innovative medical devices, the original documents should be signed and sealed by the administrative counterparts, and the Chinese documents should be signed and sealed by the agent. The "sign and seal" of the original documents means that the legal representative or the person in charge of the administrative counterparts should sign, or sign and affix the seal of the organization and should submit the notarization issued by the notary office where the administrative counterparts are located; the "sign and seal" of the Chinese documents means that the agent should affix the official seal, or the legal representative or person in charge should sign and affix the official seal. For the requirements for notarization of documents, please refer to the relevant regulations in the *Notice of the National Medical Products Administration on the Requirements for Information on Electronic Declaration of Medical Devices* (*NO.41 of 2019*).

135. Q: What is the time limit for the special review of innovative medical device and how to check the result of innovation declaration?

A: According to the relevant regulations listed in the *Special Review Procedures for Innovative Medical Devices*, after receiving the application of the special review for innovative medical device, the innovative medical device review office should issue review opinion within 60 working days (public notice and objection processing time are not counted). For the application project to be subject to special review, the administrative counterparts and the products' name should be publicized on the website of CMDE, and the publicity time should not be less than 10 working days. If there is any objection to the content of the announcement, a final review decision should be made after studying the relevant opinions. The administrative counterpart can check the review results by logging on to the review progress query page on the website of CMDE.

136. Q: What are the requirements for the provincial administration's preliminary review certification documents when the applification for special review of domestic innovative medical device is accepted for reviewing?

A: Domestic administrative counterparts should submit an application for special review of innovative medical device (the following referred to *"innovative application"*) to the provincial medical products administration where they are located. The provincial medical products administration should conduct a preliminary review on whether the application project meets the requirements of Article 2 of *The Special Review Procedures for Innovative Medical Devices*.When applying for innovation, the administrative counterparts should submit relevant supporting documents that have been initially reviewed by the provincial administration. If the innovation application have been issued an acceptance supplementary notice during the acceptance review process, and the administrative counterparts re-submit the applification after completing the supplementary issues, it is allowed not to re-carry out the provincial administation's preliminary review, and the relevant certification documents of the previous provincial administrtaion's preliminary review should be submitted as the provincial administration's preliminary review certificate. For projects that have been issued review opinions after acceptance, re-apply for the special review of innovative medical devices, they need to go through the preliminary review of the provincial administration again, and submit the relevant certification documents that have been issued during the preliminary review of the provincial administration.

137. Q: What is the time limit for the verification of the quality management system of the domestic class Ⅲ medical devices/in vitro diagnostic reagents?

A: According to the relevant regulations listed in the *Administrative Measures for Registration and Filling of Medical Device, the Administrative Measures for the Registration and Filling of In Vitro Diagnostic Reagents*, the time limit for the verification of the quality management system of domestic class Ⅲ medical devices/in vitro diagnostic reagents should be implemented in accordance with the following regulations:

(1) CMDE should notify the food and drug administrations of the corresponding provinces, autonomous regions, and municipalities to conduct verification of the registration quality management system within 10 working days from the application for registration of medical devices/in vitro diagnostic reagents.

(2) The drug supervision and administration departments of the provinces, autonomous regions and municipalities should principally

complete the verification within 30 working days after receiving the system inspection notice, and give feedback on the inspection situation, inspection results and other relevant documents to CMDE.

138. Q: What are the requirements for the sending of the verification notice and the issuance of the system verification result document of the quality management system for the registration of domestic class Ⅲ products manufactured in accordance with the medical device registrant system?

A: According to the relevant requirements in the *Notice on Further Doing a Good Job in the Pilot Program of the Class III Medical Device Registrant*, the system verification notice should be only sent to the drug supervision and administration department where the administrative counterpart (consignor) is located; The system verification result document should be sent by the local drug supervision and administration department of the administrative counterpart (consignor) to CMDE, and the system verification result report issued should indicate the name of the entrusted enterprise, manufacturing address and other information.

139. Q: If an administrative counterpart is required to participate in the expert consultation meeting, what is the participation form of the administrative counterpart?

A: According to the relevant requirements in the *Operational Specifications for Expert Consultation Meeting/Expert Public Demonstration Meeting of Center for Medical Device Evaluation. NMPA*, the participants in the expert consultation meeting are limited to the participating experts and relevant reviewers. If the administrative counterpart is required to participate in the meeting, the administrative counterpart will hold the meeting online, and the chief reviewer will summarize the questions raised at the meeting, connect the administrative counterpart through a video conference through a port, and ask the administrative counterpart to answer the questions on the spot. After the questions are answered, the administrative counterpart will exit.

140. Q: What is the time limit for the expert consultation meeting and the requirements for the avoidance time raised by the administrative counterparty?

A: According to the relevant requirements in the *Operational Specifications for Expert Consultation Meeting/Expert Public Demonstration Meeting of Center for Medical Device Evaluation. NMPA*, after the administrative counterpart receives the *Notice on Convening an Expert Consultation Meeting*, a meeting will be held within 30 working days for domestic products and 40 working days for imported products.

If there are special situations, the administrative counterpart can provide the date of avoidance from the meeting, and the date of avoidance should be within the specified time of receipt of this notice (30 working days for domestic products and 40 working days for imported products). If the avoidance time exceeds the specified time range, the administrative counterpart should file an application for extension and explain the reasons, and the application for extension should not exceed 20 working days.

141. Q: What is the agenda of the expert consultation meeting?

A: According to the relevant requirements of the *Operational Specifications for Expert Consultation Meeting/Expert Public Demonstration Meeting of Center for Medical Device Evaluation. NMPA*, the host announces the start of the meeting, and the meeting will be held according to the following agenda in principle:

(1) The personnel of the Integrated Affairs Division play the PPT video recorded by the administrative counterpart;

(2) The chief reviewer and experts discuss relevant issues, and the chief reviewer summarizes the questions;

(3) The administrative counterpart enters the venue online, the chief reviewer reads out the summary questions, the administrative counterpart makes a defense, and after the defense is over, the administrative counterpart exit the meeting;

(4) Experts review and put forward consultation opinions, and fill in the *Consultation Opinion Form for Expert Consultation Meeting*;

(5) The chief reviewer confirms that clear opinions have been obtained on the consultation questions, and assists the team leader in sorting out the joint review opinions.

142. Q: What are the conditions for CMDE to hold an expert consultation meeting during the medical device registration review?

A: According to the relevant requirements in the *Operational Specifications for Expert Consultation Meeting/Expert Public*

Demonstration Meeting of Center for Medical Device Evaluation. NMPA, if one of the following circumstances occurs, an expert consultation meeting may be held after discussion and approval by each sub-technical committee:

(1) Medical devices that have passed the innovation review;

(2) Medical devices that have passed the priority approval;

(3) Medical devices that have passed emergency approval;

(4) The first medical device of the same variety;

(5) The application for clinical trial approval.

The technical problems of other products under review should be researched and resolved by the sub-technical committees themselves. Disputes can be submitted to the central technical committee for discussion. Those who really need to consult experts can apply for an expert consultation meeting with the approval of the central technical committee.

143. Q: What are the procedures for informing the administrative counterpart prior to the expert consultation meeting?

A: According to the relevant requirements in the *Operational Specifications for Expert Consultation Meeting/Expert Public Demonstration Meeting of Center for Medical Device Evaluation. NMPA*, the procedures for informing the administrative counterpart prior to the expert consultation meeting are listed below:

(1) If the administrative counterpart is required to participate in the meeting, the Integrated Affairs Division should send the *Notice on Convening an Expert Consultation Meeting* to the administrative counterpart within 2 working days after receiving the application approval for the expert consultation meeting, and be responsible for receive the receipt. After receiving the notice, the administrative counterpart should send the receipt to the Integrated Affairs Division within 5 working days and specify in the receipt the time and reason for avoidance of the meeting, as well as the list of experts invited to participate in the meeting except for the administrative counterpart. If there are experts with conflicts of interest need to apply for avoidance, the reasons for avoidance should be specified and the real evidence should be provided.

(2) If the Integrated Affairs Division does not receive a receipt within 5 working days after sending the *Notice on Convening an Expert Consultation Meeting* to the administrative counterpart, or the Integrated Affairs Division cannot send the *Notice on Convening an Expert Consultation Meeting* due to the wrong information provided by the administrative counterpart, the Integrated Affairs Division directly arranges an expert consultation meeting within the time limit.

(3) For those who do not need the administrative counterpart to participate in the meeting, the Integrated Affairs Division directly arranges an expert consultation meeting within the time limit.

144. Q: When the national standard product is updated, under what circumstances does the registered *in vitro* diagnostic reagent need not to apply for registration change?

A: According to the management of the national standard products of in vitro diagnostic reagents by the National Institute for Food and Drug Control (hereinafter referred to as "NIFDC"), the batch number of the national standard product is composed of "variety number (6 digits) + batch number (6 digits)", which will be announced on the official website of NIFDC and can be inquired about. The update of national standard products includes two situations: "variety number change" and "batch number change". The difference is: "batch number change" is a new batch prepared to ensure the supply of national standard products. The setting, value and performance acceptance criteria of national standards have not changed, only the batch number has changed; "variety number change" means that the national standard products have totally changed, and its setting, value or performance acceptance criteria may have changed, and both the variety number and batch number have changed. Variety. Accordingly, the situation in which national standard products do not need to apply for registration change when updated include:

(1) When the batch number of the national standard product is updated during the validity period of registration certificate of medical devices (in vitro diagnostic reagents), there is no need to apply for the registration change, but relevant representation is needed in the application materials for the registration renewal.

(2) When the variety number of the national standard product is updated during the validity period of registration certificate of medical devices (in vitro diagnostic reagents), if the content of the registration certificate of registered product and its attachments have not changed, or the requirements of the new national standard product can be satisfied with the updating of the quoted variety number and batch number, there is no need to apply for the registration change. It includes the following two situations:

1) The declared product has applicable national standard

products. The product technical requirements or instructions directly quote "contents of the instructions of the national standard product" or "the national standard product variety number and batch number". The national standard product variety number and batch number have changed, and the contents of the instructions of the national standard product that quoted have not changed.

2) The declared product has no applicable national standard products. Product technical requirements or instructions refer to certain "contents of the instructions of the national standard product" or "the national standard product variety number and batch number". The national standard product variety number and batch number have changed, while the contents of the national standard product that referred to have not changed; or the contents of the national standard product have changed, but the product technical requirements or instructions still refer to the contents of the national standard products that before the change.

145. Q: If the registration applicant has no self-inspection ability at all or only part of the self-inspection ability, such as entrusting a qualified testing agency to conduct testing in whole or in part, can applicant entrust multiple qualified testing agencies to conduct testing at the same time?

A: If the registration applicant does not have the ability to inspect all or part of the items in the product technical requirements, applicants can entrust the relevant items to one or more qualified medical device inspection institutions for inspection. The registration applicant should ensure the consistency of the inspection samples that are entrusted. (For product technical requirements that fully adopt national standards or industry standards, the inspection agency must obtain the qualification certification of the national standard or industry standard, and the cover of the report should be stamped with the qualification certification mark CMA seal, and the national standards or industry standards should be indicated in the report remarks. If the inspection does not involve or partially involves national standards or industry standards, the inspection capability should be self-declared in the remarks of the inspection report, and the corresponding legal responsibility should be assumed.) When submitting a registration application, the registration applicant should form a self-inspection report according to the results of the entrusted inspection, and all the entrusted inspection reports should be submitted as attachments to the self-inspection report.

146. Q: For imported medical devices that obtained the registration certificate in China, how to apply for registration when the production is intended to be transferred from overseas to domestic?

A: According to the Notice by CMDE on the implementation of *Provisions for Medical Device Registration and Filing, Provisions for In-vitro Diagnostic Reagent Registration and Filing*, the medical devices produced in China by overseas enterprises should be registered or filed as domestic medical devices, with domestic manufacturers as applicants. For imported medical devices that obtained the registration certificate, please refer to the Announcement (No. 104 of 2020) by NMPA to submit application materials.

147. Q: For the newly established medical device manufacturers in China, can they apply for consultation on technical problems before registration when encountering technical problems during the research and development process?

A: According to Notice by CMDE, the consultation objects should be domestic medical device research and development institutions and manufacturers. Applicants with legal person certificate or business license which includes medical device production can apply for consultation on technical issues before registration is accepted.

148. Q: Can the resident representative office or office of the overseas administrative counterparty in China represent as the agent of the overseas applicant or filer?

A: According to the requirements of Article 14 of the *Administrative Measures for Registration and Filing of Medical Devices* and Article 15 of the *Administrative Measures for Registration and Filing of In Vitro Diagnostic Reagents*, overseas administrative counterparts and filing parties should designate a legal person in China as an agent, handle the registration and filing of related medical devices/in vitro diagnostic reagents. The agent should assist the administrative counterparts and the filing parties in fulfilling the obligations stipulated in the first paragraph of Article 20 of the *Regulations on the Supervision and Administration of Medical Devices*, and assist the overseas administrative counterparts and filing people to implement the corresponding legal responsibilities.

According to the above requirements, the resident representative office or office of the foreign administrative counterpart in China cannot act as an agent.

149. Q: If the administrative counterpart does not have a CA certificate, how should the relevant documents for the special review of domestic Class Ⅲ, imported Class Ⅱ, Ⅲ medical devices and innovative medical devices be submitted? How to submit the revised documents?

A: Please follow the *Announcement on the Medical Device Registration Application Materials Requirements and Approval Document Format* (*No. 121 of 2021*), *Announcement on the In Vitro Diagnostic Reagents Registration Application Materials Requirements and Approval Document Format* (*No. 122 of 2021*), and the *Announcement of the NMPA on Issuing Special Review Procedures for Innovative Medical Devices* (*No. 83 of 2018*), the regulations require that paper materials and electronic materials (content of U disk: upload data folder, folder compression package and statement of conformity) and the authorization letter of the administrative counterpart or its agent submitted by the specific applicant and a copy of their ID card are prepared and sent to Gate 3, Dacheng Plaza, No. 28, Xuanwumen West Street, Xicheng District, Beijing Window 4-7 on the first floor: 010-88331776. The staff of NMPA. will upload the documents for the administrative counterparts. After the acceptance review, if the administrative counterpart needs to make corrections, our center will send back the notice of acceptance and correction and the paper materials through EMS. If an administrative counterpart needs to re-apply after making corrections according to the acceptance opinions, it should go through the offline process. After obtaining the CA certificate, the administrative counterpart can submit the registration application, pre-review supplementary materials, and submit supplementary materials through the eRPS system. For the accepted application that was submitted offline before CA certificate came into use, it cannot be processed through the online channel of the CA certificate.

150. Q: How to effectively communicate with the acceptance hall about the accurate courier address and contact information of the acceptance notice/correction notice/filing certificate and other relevant paper materials?

A: The reception hall will give priority to the express address and contact information remarked in the "other questions that need to be explained" in the application form as the effective express information. If there is no content in this part, the applicant/ registrant/ agent information in the application form will be used as the effective express information. In order to ensure the timely and accurate delivery of relevant documents, it is recommended to fill in the registration application form accurately.

151. Q: How to judge the time to apply for renewal of registration is 6 months before the expiration of the medical device registration certificate?

A: If the medical device registration certificate needs to be renewed after the expiration of the validity period, the registrant should apply for the renewal of registration 6 months before the expiration of the medical device registration certificate, and follow the submit application materials as required. If the application materials are incomplete or do not conform to the statutory form and need to be supplemented and corrected, our center will indicate the time of the registrant's first application for renewal of registration in the notification of acceptance of corrections. When the registrant applies for renewal of registration again after making corrections, he should submit the notice of acceptance of supplements and corrections. The Center For medical Device Evaluation. NMPA will determine whether the application for renewal of registration is within 6 months after the expiration of the validity period of the medical device registration certificate according to the time of the registrant's first application for renewal of registration indicated in the notice of acceptance of supplements and corrections, and review the application materials in accordance with the provisions of the *Administrative Measures for Registration and Filing of Medical Devices.*

152. Q: When the content of the mandatory standards cited in the technical requirements of registered medical devices (IVD) products has changed, under what circumstances is there no need to apply for change registration?

A: If new mandatory standards are released and implemented within the validity period of the medical device (IVD) registration certificate, the registration certificate of registered products and the items specified in their attachments could meet the new mandatory standards without any changes, including the following two situations:

(1) The declared product has applicable mandatory standards. Product technical requirements refer to mandatory standards in the

form of "directly citing the specific content of mandatory standard clauses" , "standard number" or "standard number + year number" . The mandatory standard is updated, the standard number and/or year number is changed, while the content of the mandatory standard clause referenced in the technical requirements of the product remains unchanged.

(2) There is no applicable mandatory standard for the declared product. The technical requirements of the product refer to the terms of a mandatory standard, the mandatory standard is updated, the standard number and/or the year number has changed, while the content of the standard terms the technical requirements refer to has not changed; or the content of the mandatory standard terms referenced the product technical requirements has changed, but the product technical requirements still refer to the mandatory standard terms before the update.

In the above two cases, the technical requirements of the product do not need to be changed or only to be changed by the standard number and/or standard year number, and no change registration is required.

153. Q: Is the *Chinese Pharmacopoeia* considered as a mandatory standard for medical devices? The performance indicators and inspection methods of "sterility" in the product technical requirements have already met the 2015 version of the *Chinese Pharmacopoeia*. Do they need to be upgraded to comply with the 2020 version of the *Chinese Pharmacopoeia*?

A: The *Chinese Pharmacopoeia* is not a mandatory standard for medical devices. If the product has applicable mandatory standards, and the mandatory standard refers to the *Chinese Pharmacopoeia* without indicating the version number. If the registrant needs to update the content of the *Chinese Pharmacopoeia* in the product technical requirements to the 2020 version, it is necessary to apply for change registration , and then apply for renewal of registration after obtaining the change document; if the product has applicable mandatory standards, and the mandatory standard refers to the *Chinese Pharmacopoeia* with a clear version number of 2015, or the *Chinese Pharmacopoeia* cited in the sterility test is not quoted in mandatory standards, or the product has no mandatory standard, it can be renewed without change with referring to the 2015 version of the *Chinese Pharmacopoeia*.

154. Q: When applying for renewal of registration, if there is no change in a registered medical device (IVD) product itself, only the mandatory standards applicable to the product are updated, can registrant submit a test report that meets the new mandatory standards?

A: If the mandatory citation of registration renewal involves the change of its specific terms, it is recommended to submit the application for registration change separately and obtain the registration change document approved by the original approval department before submitting the application for registration renewal. However, the registrant should apply for renewal of registration 6 months before the expiration of the medical device registration certificate, and submit application materials in accordance with relevant requirements. If the application materials are incomplete or do not conform to the statutory form and need to be supplemented and corrected, our center will indicate the time of the registrant's first application for renewal of registration in the notification of acceptance of supplements and corrections. When the registrant applies for renewal of registration again after making corrections, he should submit a notice of acceptance of supplements and corrections. CMDE will determine whether the application for renewal of registration is within 6 months before the expiration of the validity period of the medical device registration certificate according to the time of the registrant's first application for renewal of registration indicated in the notice of acceptance of supplements and corrections, and review the application materials in accordance with the provisions of the *Administrative Measures for Registration and Filing of Medical Devices* or the *Measures for the Administration of Registration and Filing of In Vitro Diagnostic Reagents*.

155. Q: The owner of the main document of the medical device or its agent needs to use the CA (Certificate Authority) to register the main document. How to prepare the CA application data?

A: As of March 15, 2021, when applying for a CA, the domestic master document owner or the agent entrusted by the import master document owner in China must prepare the *Medical Device Master Document Registration Application Form* to be submitted on the master document registration platform at the same time. After being sealed by the applicant, it will be uploaded together with the business license to the "1.5 Scanning Copy of Enterprise Business License" section of the "CA Certificate Application" module.

156. Q: If the system prompts that the CA certificate is about to expire, what should administrative counterpart need to do?

A: The validity period of the CA certificate after the first application is one year. When the validity period of the CA certificate is less than 60 days, the system will prompt that the certificate is about to expire. If the administrative counterpart wants to continue to use the CA certificate, he/she should insert the CA into the computer before CA is out of period of validity and log in to the official website of CMDE (https://erps.cmde.org.cn). Click "Certificate Renewal and Update" and operate according to the prompts on the web page to extend the validity period for one year. For the specific operation process, please see the *Notice on Issues Related to the Renewal of the Digital Authentication Certificate of the Electronic Declaration Information System for Medical Device Registration* on the website of CMDE.

157. Q: Can the administrative counterpart confirm the contents of the medical device registration certificate or the change document before it is officially issued, so as to reduce the error of the information contained in the registration certificate and the attachment?

A: Yes. Before formally issuing the registration certificate or change document, CMDE will ask the administrative counterpart to confirm the contents of the registration certificate or change document and its attachments (product technical requirements, instructions, registration certificate or change document information in the form of attached pages).

For online projects, CMDE will send the *Medical Device Registration Certificate Information Confirmation Form* (the followingreferred to as the Confirmation Form) containing the registration certificate or change document information of the corresponding project and the attachment of the registration certificate or change document to the administrative counterpart through the eRPS system. The administrative counterpart will log in to the eRPS system with the CA to receive the Confirmation Form, view the content to be confirmed for the corresponding project and verify it item by item. After all the information has been confirmed, click the "Finish Confirmation" button to reply to the confirmation result. If the contents of the attachment are incorrect, the administrative counterpart is also requested to send the PDF file of the final version of the attachment after confirmation to the reviewer's email. The offline project will issue the "Confirmation Form" by e-mail. For detailed operation, please refer to the *Notice on Confirmation of Medical Device Registration Certificate and its Annex Information* issued by CMDE.

158. Q: If the administrative counterpart finds that the received registration certificate, change document and its attachments have contents that need to be corrected, and the contents are not substantive changes, the original registration application data can fully support the authenticity, accuracy and rationality of the correction. In this case, which preferred correction method should administrative counterpart choose?

A: The administrative counterpart can go to the Certification

Office of the Administrative Affairs Acceptance Service and Complaint Reporting Center of NMPA, explain the situation to the staff of the Certification Office and apply for the amendment of the registration certificate information. At the same time, apply for a *Registration Certificate Information Confirmation Application Form*, completethe "filled in by the applicant" part of the form, and return it to the staff of the Certification Office after signing or sealing. After receiving the form, the corresponding chief examiner of CMDE will judge the amended contents and hand the results back to the Certification Office at the first time. The administrative counterpart will wait for the notification of the Certification Office, and then receive the amended registration certificate or change documents and attachments.

159. Q: Will CMDE inform the administrative counterpart of the review conclusion to be rejected and provide the opportunity to raise objectionsduring the review of the application for registration of medical devices?

A: Before the formal issuance of the rejected review conclusion, CMDE will inform the administrative counterpart of the conclusion and reason of the rejection by pushing the *Confirmation Form of the Rejected Conclusion of the Medical Device Registration Technical Review* (here referred to as the Confirmation Form). If the administrative counterpart has any objection, it should raise it within 15 working days from the date of receiving the confirmation form, If no objection is raised within 15 working days, it shall be deemed as agreeing with the conclusion and reason of disapproval. For online application projects, push and confirm the Confirmation